FIT, FIERCE, AND FABULOUS OVER 50!

THE SECRET TO LIFELONG HEALTH, ENERGY, AND WEIGHT MANAGEMENT THROUGH ANTI-INFLAMMATORY INTERMITTENT FASTING FOR WOMEN

KARIN FELTMAN, RN

CONTENTS

DISCLAIMER

Medical Disclaimer: This book is not a medical guide. You are advised to consult a medical professional before implementing any drastic lifestyle changes, including diet, supplements, and physical exercise. Do not discontinue the use of medication unless instructed by your healthcare provider.

Trigger Warning: The information in this book may be a trigger and should be undertaken with caution. If you have a history of disordered eating and find yourself going down an unhealthy path as you read about or adopt this lifestyle, please stop immediately and seek help. The purpose of this book is to bring dietary freedom, so feelings contrary to this should be noted and processed before proceeding.

INTRODUCTION

Know that you are the perfect age. Each year is special and precious, for you shall only live it once. Be comfortable with growing older.

— LOUISE HAY

- Are you feeling lost and frustrated with the changes happening within your body?
- Are you constantly fatigued, with no energy or enthusiasm?
- Are you feeling disheartened because you have been sitting on that weight plateau for longer than you'd care to admit?

- Are you tiptoeing your way into menopause and afraid of what's to come?
- Are you an empty-nester who has spent years focusing on caring for others and now find yourself hovering in limbo without a solid identity and not sure how to care for yourself?

These are just a handful of the questions that many women ask themselves when they reach certain milestones in their lives. Think about your life—where you have been and where you currently find yourself. I have just one question: Are you ready to step out of the shadows to claim your spotlight, front and center in your life? This book can show you how.

I would like to personally welcome you to this journey, where you will learn how to reclaim your health and well-being. As you can see by the title—Fit, Fierce, and Fabulous Over 50!—this book is dedicated to everyone who is edging towards or has already crossed the barrier into their 50s. We have all heard that "age is just a number," but with the number 50 comes unique challenges and considerations. This age (and every age thereafter) can be glorious if you have the key to unlocking optimal health and holistic wellness at any age. That is what we will be exploring together.

My vision for this book is to allow everyone to claim a starting point to join this journey. You get to set the pace. I am here to encourage you, give you the motivation you need, equip you with helpful information, and provide practical and valuable tools to make this transition easier. I will also share some personal stories to show you how I walked this road before you. Let's get started!

ROADMAP TO RECLAIMING YOUR "FIT, FIERCE, AND FABULOUS"

I can assure you that this is not a book that will shame you into changing the way you eat, drink, exercise, think, or anything else. I believe that everyone has the right to make their own choices based on a combination of factual information and what they feel is right for them. I won't tell you to box all of your candy, cookies, chips, and cereals and toss them in the trash—unless you want to. This book will take you back to the beginning and teach you the basic ground rules. Everyone knows that babies need to learn how to roll over before they can sit, they need to sit before they can crawl, they need to crawl before they can walk, and walk before they can run. This is also the best way to approach a lifestyle change—first things first, and one step at a time.

This book may be geared toward women, but I believe that it should be read by everyone regardless of gender, age, ethnicity, or the multitude of hats they wear and the roles they play. Everyone knows someone struggling, and what better way to show compassion than to walk alongside them as they travel the road to healing? It is time to take a look at the roadmap to see what can be expected on this journey. I will help equip you with the tools you need to reclaim control over your physical and mental health and well-being. This path is not going to be easy, but the wealth of knowledge and information will help light the way forward until you can see light at the end of your own tunnel.

The Highlights of Your Impending Journey

Experience has taught me that people are in a hurry to reach their goals without understanding the unique dynamics that will get them there and help maintain them. That is what I want this book to be for you—a guide to understanding the ins and outs of an intermittent fasting lifestyle and information to help you maintain this lifestyle and the benefits that go with it for a lifetime. This is not a race to see who can lose the most weight or get to their goals the fastest. This is about identifying, modifying, correcting, and assisting you to find your "fit, fierce, and fabulous" before, during, and after you reach the big 5-0. Let's look at a quick breakdown of what's to come.

Eating Habits

A cautionary look at the dangers of disordered eating, especially when making drastic changes to your lifestyle. We will explore who should not participate in intermittent fasting or other types of restricted eating and the warning signs of falling into disordered eating patterns. We will look at the difference between disordered eating and eating disorders, as well as resources for those believing they need help and support.

Exploring Intermittent Fasting

Nearly everyone has an opinion about intermittent fasting, and rarely are those opinions backed up by solid facts or research. There is a lot of misinformation and myth surrounding IF, and we will sort out fact from fiction. It would be unfair and unjustified to dismiss the idea of intermittent fasting because it didn't work for someone else—no two people or bodies are the same. I would encourage you to tune out the stories from others about how intermittent fasting failed them and instead take this challenge: If you decide to incorporate the intermittent fasting strategy into your lifestyle, commit to giving it a full 30-day trial before you pass judgment. I believe 30 days gives you time to adjust to the changes, modify the strategy to suit your lifestyle, and see results.

We will be introduced to 10 different methods of intermittent fasting and the pros and cons of each. You will be given the information you need to choose the best fit for your goals and lifestyle needs.

The Great Weight Loss Revelation

No two people or bodies are the same. You cannot measure your progress based on someone else's journey. Weight loss is individual to each person. Lifestyle changes will affect each individual differently, so it's best not to enter into a "competition" with others to see who can lose the most weight in a set period of time. That sets you up for discouragement if your progress does not match your partner's. This is something everyone needs to learn and understand, and it is essential that you don't give up because of disappointment. Remember that you are unique in every way, shape, and form—you don't have to achieve the same goals as someone else to be successful. Reaching optimal weight can also take time, and your body often needs a time of transition before fully responding to a change in lifestyle. Give it the time it needs, and focus on non-scale victories and clues to evaluate how IF is working for you.

The Big Five-Oh Expectation

What can you expect when you hit 50 and beyond? This chapter touches on physical, mental, and emotional issues specific to both age and gender and how intermittent fasting can help with each.

Exercise

This is a topic everyone loves to hate. I will not tell you to join a gym, but I will say that physical exercise is an excellent companion for intermittent fasting. If you are hesitant to work out in public, your home offers you a safe space to get in the movement you need to stay healthy. You can join online communities that offer fitness or yoga classes, do videos at your own pace, crank up your favorite playlist and dance, or get in a cardio workout while vigorously sweeping or mopping your floor.

We will examine how exercise and intermittent fasting interact and special considerations for incorporating exercise into your IF routine. I will also give some tips for combating common challenges experienced when combining exercise and restricted eating.

A Note From Me

I know this change may seem intimidating, but I can assure you that the transition will be painless with the right amount of information, knowledge, and guidance. You get to set the pace during your transition period, which will help you manage your expectations and find your way to your own version of fit, fierce, and fabulous. Hey, if I could do it —anyone can.

Food Stuff

Though IF is more about when to eat than what to eat, its benefits can be maximized by including an anti-inflammatory way of eating. I will give you information on what an anti-inflammatory diet is and the benefits of eating this way. We will discuss the ins and outs of meal planning, prepping, and shopping, and I will give you a sample weekly meal plan and 50 delicious, plant-based recipes to get you started.

Tips and Tricks

Knowledge is power, but we also need practical tools and ideas to make a lifestyle change that will stick. We will learn about the best way to maintain your IF while socializing, ways to track your progress, and support resources so that you don't feel like you are in this alone.

THE ROAD TO MY OWN FIT, FIERCE, AND FABULOUS OVER 50!

I always loved my birthday. It was the highlight of my year. I would start celebrating a month in advance and drop not-so-subtle reminders to everyone I knew that my birthday was approaching. I used to plan my day in detail, which would entail visiting various places around town that gave out an assortment of freebies on your big day. I would grab a friend, and we would have a complimentary breakfast, free specialty coffees, a barbecue lunch, and a movie with soda and popcorn. We would also indulge in free ice creams and take a movie rental home for the next day. After turning 21, I could get a free drink at the local nightclub, where I danced the night away with friends. This was a tradition for me, and I spent 364 days a year looking forward to it. To make the day even more special, my friend and I would usually enjoy a day at the spa and then enjoy a luxurious dinner at a high-end restaurant afterward. Yes, I loved my birthday— until I hit the big Five-Oh.

I detested my 50th birthday. I had started dreading it months in advance because that number hit me as no other had in the past. I hated it with a passion, and I was embarrassed by it. It wasn't just the number I hated; in all honesty, it was the inward reflection of what this milestone forced me to see. I detested the person that looked back at me from the mirror. I didn't recognize her because I disliked who I had become. How did this happen? How did the changes come on so rapidly? Truth be told, I know that the transformation occurred gradually, and I could track the progression. I may have been in denial, but turning 50 caused me to look at myself head-on. I became someone I never thought or imagined would look back at me from the mirror. I didn't recognize myself in the reflection.

I didn't feel fit, fierce, or fabulous. I had gained a lot of weight. My skin had lost its glow. My hair, once my crowning glory, was dull, drab, boring, and out of style. I couldn't find the sparkle in my eye—it had gone into hiding. My personality reflected my outward appearance. I had lost the vitality and joy I had always incorporated into my life. I lost my humor, my sense of adventure, and the light in my soul had dimmed. I was out of shape, out of ideas, and I was out of hope. I wanted to crawl into a hole and avoid being noticed. I was okay with just existing because I didn't want anyone looking at me and judging me the way I judged myself. I couldn't imagine what this meant for my life moving forward into my 50s, much less beyond.

The Turnaround

I can only thank God for those friends I previously mentioned. My friend Paula appeared on my doorstep on my ill-fated birthday. She had a look of determination on her face—armed with a shiny plastic bedazzled princess crown and sash—and dragged me away from my pity party. She helped me get ready for my "special day" and insisted that we follow the previous years' traditions, including a visit to the spa and the addition of a session in a float tank—this is a story for later.

We visited all the places that offered freebies, enjoyed drinks and a fancy dinner, and lived in the moment. I was able to see myself through her eyes when I was in her presence. I regained some sense of the "old" me that had gone into hiding. I saw myself through a new lens and rediscovered the person that was missing—me. I did have fun on my 50th birthday. It was an eye-opening day and a revelation that I could say goodbye to the "old" me and begin to discover a new identity. That was when I decided to start working on a new and improved version of myself. I realized that age has no hold over me and shouldn't prevent me from reaching my goals. I began to believe—to know—that I could become the best me I could be, at any age! As I write this, I am 54 years old. I am more fabulous now than I was at any other age. Guess what? You can be, too.

It Can Be Done

How did I do it? It started with resolve. I wouldn't have accomplished anything if I didn't have determination. The first step on this new journey was deciding what I wanted to change. I decided I needed to be kind and gentle with myself and treat myself with the grace and respect I deserve. I believe you have to take baby steps to love yourself, and you can achieve that by getting to know yourself again. Speak to yourself in the mirror, and tell yourself how wonderful and amazing you are. Loving yourself into a better state of mind is more effective than hating yourself into it.

Life is a choice, and I choose to embrace the small changes. I celebrate my successes instead of making all-or-nothing commitments. I don't leave any openings for despair and failure that could potentially present setbacks. I change the less-than-healthy parts of my life, especially regarding my dietary choices and physical activity levels. I make conscious decisions based on what is right for me.

The first changes involved adding healthy activities and choices that aligned with my fitness levels at that time. My food choices included items I could tweak or swap for something more nutritious. I gradually packed the less-healthy options into trash bags and got rid of them. I took my time and set a pace that was comfortable for me. I treated myself to a visit to the salon and got a cut, color, and blowout. I bought myself a new outfit—one that was flattering and made me feel good about myself. My attitude changed, and I acknowledged that every day is a new day. I realized that I had a choice concerning every aspect of my health moving forward. All I had to do was accept who I am, realize that I am in control, and live each day to the maximum.

The two biggest factors in my transformation and revitalization were my decision to adopt a more anti-inflammatory plant-based way of eating and include intermittent fasting into my lifestyle. The combination of the two has had a profound effect on my health, my looks, my energy levels, and my outlook on the future. I cannot recommend the combination of anti-inflammatory and intermittent fasting lifestyles more highly. You can follow one without the other and still see the results, but I am leaving the decision up to you. This is not an all-or-nothing lifestyle, and you have the freedom to choose how to apply it to your life and situation. If you are hesitant about eating plants or worried about confining yourself to a restrictive eating window, stick with me until the end before making your final decision. I am confident you can use this information to make an informed decision about what is best for you. No one knows your situation better than you do, and you can still positively impact your weight, your health, and your life. You've got this!

1

NOT SO FAST—A WORD OF CAUTION

- Are you prepared to work on your relationship with your body?
- Are you ready to repair the relationship that you have with food?
- Are you willing to explore the mind/body connection and what that means for you in terms of eating?

Eating is perhaps the most fundamental activity on earth. We all need to do it in some form. Yet it is also SOOOO complicated. The experience is as unique as each individual. Some can eat whatever they want, whenever they want, and not gain an ounce. Their bodies seem naturally perfect. Others eat until they are stuffed yet are unable to gain precious pounds, despite being skin and bones. Some see a slice of cake or smell pizza and instantly gain weight. No matter the struggle, the struggle is real.

No one will ever fully understand the silent battle that is being waged between another person and their food. This complicated relationship can, if left unchecked, lead to various types of disordered eating. Society has placed absolute judgment on what is and isn't healthy, both in terms of food and body types, and often conveys that publicly through comments or stares. This type of judgment and abuse can cause people to eat in secret, away from the prying eyes of others, and lead to unhealthy food behaviors.

Intermittent fasting is meant to lead to freedom from, and a solution for, obsession with food. Eating within a set window frees up time often spent focused on food when eating all day long. Though intermittent fasting is typically accompanied by healthy eating for best results, it also allows for more flexibility and grace to eat your favorite foods than more restrictive "diets." IF is not a diet; it is a lifestyle—one designed to alleviate anxiety associated with food, body weight, and health, as it addresses all of those at once. We will go into specifics in future chapters, but first, we must work on mindset.

THE COMPLICATED RELATIONSHIP BETWEEN YOU, YOUR FOOD, AND YOUR BODY

Disordered eating is a serious physical and mental condition that affects over 65% of women in the United States. A team of doctors and specialists at the University of North Carolina in Chapel Hill conducted a survey in 2008 in which 4,023 women participated in a study regarding their dietary habits. They were women aged 25 to 45, and 65% reported that they have had or were currently struggling with disordered eating. This is the reality we are facing when it comes to our relationship with food. Additionally, 10% of the women reportedly suffered from diagnosed eating disorders such as bulimia nervosa, binge eating, or anorexia. This means that a staggering 75% of women were struggling with eating habits that negatively affected their relationship with food and their bodies (University of North Carolina at Chapel Hill, 2008).

The Symptoms of Disordered Eating

I believe that the most common symptom of disordered eating is shame. Shame over our bodies, surrounding our irregular eating habits, and shame over the lack of control that everyone else seems to have when it comes to food. More than 9% of people worldwide have a diagnosed eating disorder, and countless others have disordered eating, so that puts those of us with disordered eating in good company. It is important to get past the shame and overcome our embarrassment to seek help and begin healing before our physical and emotional health is permanently affected.

Although disordered eating and eating disorders are different, they are similar, and both have devastating effects on our physical, mental, and emotional health. Disordered eating is any irregular eating pattern that doesn't fall under a specific eating disorder diagnosis. This can include obsession with dieting, emotional overeating, food restriction as self-punishment, and even a regimented compulsion to eat a "clean" or healthy diet. Basically, unhealthy thoughts or practices surrounding food would be considered disordered eating.

Disordered eating is more common than many want to acknowledge, and I believe it is something that many suffer from without realizing it. While eating disorders affect at least 9% of people worldwide, it is harder to estimate the number of people with disordered eating because it is difficult to classify and often goes untreated. The media and culture play a significant role in steering people down the road to eating disorders, as advertisements promote products with unattainable results, and photoshopped models portray unrealistic ideals. Celebrity endorsements and social media influencers promise amazing results with zero effort, and we scramble to follow one fad after another in an attempt to finally realize our goals.

This desperation to reach our goals through whatever means necessary leads people to develop an unhealthy relationship with food and a hatred for their imperfect bodies. This causes disordered eating patterns, which, if left unchecked, open the doors for the development of a full-blown eating disorder. Disordered eating, as well as eating disorders, can have devastating effects not only on the person suffering from them but also on families, friends, and loved ones. I want to help you discover how to love your body, love the food that powers your body, and claim that spotlight that will showcase your fit, fierce, and fabulous self!

Here is a list of some of the most common disordered eating symptoms and behaviors. These are symptoms that have either been shared with me by others or ones that I have experienced myself. Read through each one carefully, and see which ones resonate with you. This is meant to be a tool to help recognize where you, or someone you love, may currently be struggling. Remember—no shame! This is merely a jumping-off point to identify whether or not you need help in this area.

- You exercise excessively to lose weight.
- You exercise obsessively to prevent weight gain.
- A large part of your day is centered around meal planning, prep, cooking, and eating.
- You are always on a diet.
- You jump from diet to diet when you don't achieve the desired results.
- You feel guilty when you nibble on a cookie or lick your fingers after touching a piece of chocolate.

- You are a secret eater.
- You label food as "good" or "bad" based on your eating plan.
- You rigidly restrict yourself from eating certain foods because they are "not good" for you.
- You eat (or restrict eating) in response to your emotions. This could be for comfort, to relieve stress and anxiety, or even in times of celebration.
- You will purposefully skip meals, even when hungry.
- You weigh daily (or more) and obsess over the number on the scale, including small fluctuations.
- You eat everything in sight and have little to no restraint when it comes to overeating.
- You use restrictive measures such as excessive exercising, water intake, or fasting to compensate for eating a "bad" or off-limits food.
- You experience unregulated body temperatures.
- You turn down invitations to social events, family get-togethers, or nights out with friends for fear that you may have to eat in front of a crowd.
- You will cook food but not participate in enjoying the meal, feigning that cooking calms your appetite.
- You find yourself overeating so that you can induce vomiting to help you cleanse your stomach.
- You make use of medications or practices such as laxatives or enemas to ensure your intestines are clear of any residual foods.

- You use appetite suppressants or diet tablets to prevent you from eating.
- You use whatever method you can to control or lose weight, regardless of the health consequences.
- You feel that you are fat, despite being underweight on traditional measurement charts.

The Harmful Side Effects of Disordered Eating

As I read through the list of symptoms, my heart breaks for everyone struggling with disordered eating. This is a silent and lonely disease that needs a voice. That is why I felt led to write this book—to share my story and help others find their health and happiness. We all deserve to feel good in our bodies and confident in our skin—regardless of our shape or size.

Let's take a look at what disordered eating can do to our bodies and why it is so important to heal our relationship with food.

Disordered eating has a real chance of progressing to full-blown eating disorders such as bulimia or anorexia, which can not only have devastating effects on health but can also be deadly.

- Drastically restricting your food intake will deprive you of the necessary nutrients that your body needs to do things like healing and protecting your bones.

- You need the sustenance that only food can provide to ensure you enjoy a good night's rest; without the necessary nutrients, you will be lethargic and suffer from insomnia.
- Excessive use of medication or food deprivation will lead to stomach problems such as ulcers, diarrhea, or constipation.
- You run the risk of suffering from chronic headaches that may affect your ability to think or work.
- Scale watchers may find themselves experiencing guilt, shame, and feelings of failure when the numbers don't work in their favor.
- Disordered eating opens a door that can lead us down the dark passages of depression, anxiety, and low self-esteem.
- Severe calorie restriction leads to nutrient deficiencies and inefficient metabolism.
- Other adverse side effects include electrolyte imbalances, dehydration, erratic heart rate, blood pressure issues, and more.

BEEN THERE, DONE THAT! YOU ARE NOT ALONE

I know all about eating disorders—more accurately, I know all about having eating disorders. This is something that I have been struggling with since I was a young girl. For as long as I can remember, I have been battling a health disorder that went undiagnosed until I turned 50. This disorder, Lipedema, affected the size and shape of my legs, butt, and upper arms, and it spiraled me into a battle with myself that I couldn't win. The expectations of society and the media had me wanting to be like those women portrayed as "perfect" and "normal" in magazines and on television. The harder I tried to be the replica of what I saw, the more I came to believe I was failing. In my mind, I was neither "perfect" nor "normal."

It didn't take long to develop an addiction to exercise. Believing the lies that I was eating too much and not exercising enough, I turned to countless hours in the gym, hoping I had found my savior. While I could feel my muscles growing underneath the layer of fat that remained above, I wasn't making much progress toward my goal. In fact, the increasing muscle mass made me look larger than before. Further spiraling down into feelings of failure and shame, I turned to diet. I was prepared to go to the extreme, including starving myself. I started counting calories—everything I ate was accounted for, even vitamins and medication. I refused to consume more than 500 calories a day. I would even go as far as chewing my food and spitting it out before swallowing it. All I wanted was the satisfaction of enjoying the taste but I was terrified of the consequences of eating. I found myself completely ensnared in anorexia, but it wasn't enough.

My anorexia turned into bulimia as time progressed. I would eat, then sneak away to purge everything I had just eaten. I did this regardless of how much or how little I had consumed. I was desperate to be thin! My legs and butt were not responding. I still didn't resemble the models I saw in the advertisements in magazines or on TV and billboards. This was especially painful and humiliating because I was a model —from age 13 until my early-to-mid 20s. From the first day, I was told that I was beautiful, but—the dreaded "but"—I needed to lose weight. I had a pretty face, but... I needed to work on my size. Keep in mind that at the time, I was six feet tall and weighed a mere 145 pounds. I began to see myself in a distorted way and developed body dysmorphia—a mental health condition that has an obsessive focus on actual or perceived flaws in the body. In other words, when I looked in the mirror, that was all I could see. Flaws.

I had let society and others determine who and how I should be. I forgot where my true identity came from—God and deep within myself. I had forgotten the things that truly made me valuable, such as my character and my heart of compassion. I allowed external influences to become internal values, which nearly cost me my life. It wasn't until I began to realize these things that the road to healing could truly begin.

I won't lie. I still struggle with body issues today. I still have the occasional urge to restrict food, do a crash diet, or the desire to vomit when I have had too much to eat. Those are wounds that run deep and may never be fully healed. I know my worth, and I know what is important. I no longer judge myself by anyone else's standards. I focus on what is right with me and not what is "wrong" or "flawed." Each morning, I set the intention to be the best me possible and to walk in health. I am physically, emotionally, mentally, relationally, and spiritually in the best place I have ever been. Fit, fierce, and fabulous have nothing to do with being a body-beautiful or skinny woman—they have everything to do with being authentic versions of our beautiful selves. Guess what? That is one goal we can and will achieve if we set our minds to it.

The Road to Treatment and Help

- Are you ready to admit that you have a problem?
- Are you ready to take back what has been taken from you?

Do you suspect that you may be suffering from disordered eating? Reach out to someone you trust, and share your suspicions with them. A true friend will not dismiss your feelings and can help you search for someone who specializes in eating disorders. A qualified therapist and dietician will guide you in rebuilding your trust and relationship with food. Doing this is paramount to your healing journey, as well as crucial to the success of adopting any healthy eating lifestyle. Other resources include in-person support groups such as Overeaters Anonymous or a variety of free and paid online support communities that are just an internet search away. If you are not comfortable seeking out these resources, start by talking with your healthcare provider for their recommendation.

We live in a world where it is common to condemn others for being less than our perception of "perfect." Eating disorders and disordered eating have most likely been around since the day someone first developed a "diet" or said, "You should lose some weight." This has spiraled us into something no one could have foreseen: self-harm on a massive scale. It is time to turn our back on the lies and follow the truth in pursuit of our fit, fierce, and fabulous!

Let's get up close and personal with intermittent fasting. IF is not a diet but a lifestyle. We will start by debunking some of the most common myths and misconceptions about intermittent fasting. Buckle up—it's going to be quite a ride!

2

DEBUNKING MYTHS ABOUT INTERMITTENT FASTING

E veryone seems to have an opinion on all things health-related and is quick to share whenever you try to adopt a new, healthy lifestyle. It's hard to blame them, as misinformation is everywhere. In this day and age, people are gaining knowledge from social media platforms, blog posts, and their friends' Facebook pages. Unable to weed out fact from fiction, they are armed with misinformation and ready to pass that on to you. That usually comes in the form of negativity or discouragement.

It is essential to understand that fasting is more than just a catchphrase or craze invented by someone to make a buck. The history of fasting predates all of us. It is used for much more than just weight loss. For instance, physicians advise their patients to fast for up to eight hours before surgery or invasive procedures. Others have their patients fast or restrict calories during cancer treatment, to increase the effectiveness of chemotherapy. There are many uses for fasting, some medical and some not. Let's take a look.

FUN AND HISTORICAL FACTS ABOUT FASTING

Fasting is practiced in some form by nearly all of the world's major religions, including Christianity, Hinduism, Buddhism, and Islam. Devout Muslims participate in a month-long fast called Ramadan. During this time, they abstain from eating or drinking from sunrise to sunset for a period of thirty days or until the new moon has been sighted. This is to help bring to mind those in need and to practice thankfulness. Christians fast for multiple reasons. Some fast for periods ranging from one to forty days to seek clarity and guidance from God or an answer to specific prayers. Others observe a forty-day period of fasting from specific foods or practices, called Lent, in remembrance of Jesus' forty days of temptation in the desert, where he abstained from consuming food and water. Fasting is also a regular part of many Hindu and Buddhist religious festivals.

Fasting has been used as part of medical therapy dating back to the fifth century. It is believed that Hippocrates, the Greek physician, restricted the food and beverages of his patients when they showed signs of ailments. This was also adopted by other doctors who noted that sick patients naturally declined to consume food because they had no appetite when sick with certain illnesses (Migala, 2022). In other words, fasting was not only prescribed by physicians but also naturally adopted by patients themselves, who intuitively abstained from food when ill.

An Introduction to the Intermittent Fasting Phenomenon

Fasting has been around since the beginning of time. Nearly everyone has knowingly participated in fasting at some point in their life, but all of us unconsciously fast as well—at night! Each night (or day, depending on your work schedule), as you sleep, your body goes into a state of rest and fasting, allowing your organs to work their magic as they break down food and drinks you've consumed during the day and disperse their nutrients throughout your body. After digestion is complete, your body goes into a state of healing, repairing damage, and clearing out toxins. Fasting is not only healthy; it is one of our body's built-in maintenance mechanisms.

The term "intermittent fasting" is relatively new. It was first introduced to the general public in 2012 by Dr. Michael Mosley, a BBC journalist who wanted to lose weight and become healthy without disrupting his lifestyle. He produced the documentary *Eat, Fast, and Live Longer* in an attempt to perfect the fine art of fasting. He has also written multiple books, and *The Fast Diet* is credited with introducing the intermittent fasting lifestyle to billions of individuals. This flung the doors wide open for other authors to share their versions of IF and what worked for them (Tello, 2018).

That is what this book is—my version. I did not invent intermittent fasting. I am not the topmost expert in the field. While I have done extensive research, I am not the one with the most profound knowledge of the physiology behind how it works. Many others have gone before and laid that foundation—and I am eternally grateful to them. I want to refer you to books by experts like Gin Stephens and Dr. Jason Fung for the full science behind IF. Instead, this is my story. The story of coming face-to-face with the demons of weight and chronic illness and coming out the other side victorious. It is the story of learning to love myself and the skin I'm in through intermittent fasting. It is the story of my road to being fit, fierce, and fabulous! Join me.

THE TRUTH AND THE LIES

People love to hear good news about their bad habits. They are willing to believe anything that tells them they don't need to change or that achieving good health is easy. The truth is, I'd love to believe that too! They will try to knock you off your path, especially if it is threatening to them. After all, if you succeed, they will have to take action because knowledge is power. As a result, lots of self-serving myths about IF abound.

In the world of intermittent fasting, like in all things, there is lots of "fake news." But the truth is, well… true. So, let's try to sort it out.

The Fad Phenomenon

I have heard intermittent fasting called a "fad" and a "crash diet." The truth is, it is neither. According to the dictionary, the definition of a fad is an intense and widely shared enthusiasm for something, especially one that is short-lived and without basis in the object's qualities; a craze. While there is undoubtedly widespread enthusiasm for IF, it has proven to be much more than a short-lived craze. As we saw in our "fun facts," it has been around for at least thousands of years! The enthusiasm for IF is due to its effectiveness and ability to bring healing. That's far from a fad.

A crash diet is one in which a person loses a lot of weight quickly through drastic calorie reduction (800–1200 calories/day). When done in a healthy manner, neither of these things is true with IF. Intermittent fasting focuses on when to eat and neither mandates nor advises a drastic calorie restriction. If an individual needs to lose weight, approximately 500 calories below the amount needed to maintain weight is suggested. This will allow for one pound a week of fat loss. Intermittent fasting can be used for both weight loss and healthy weight maintenance, but rapid weight reduction is neither the standard nor the goal.

The bottom line is this—fasting has not only been around for thousands of years but will likely continue to play a role in people's lives for thousands of years to come. The addition of the word "intermittent" may have caused some confusion and contributed to the misconception that IF is a "diet" rather than a way of eating. When done correctly and with the right intentions, though, it is beneficial to overall physical health and mental well-being. You are in control of this lifestyle—not the other way around. You get to set the rules and do what works for you. More on that later!

Flex Those Muscles

One of the biggest pushbacks I get in terms of intermittent fasting is the concern that it will lead to muscle loss. There is the belief that during fasting time, especially if combining IF with exercise, the body will burn muscle for fuel. The fear is that this will lead to muscle damage and loss. Others claim that the body won't get adequate protein to build muscle if done in conjunction with a diet low in animal proteins and high in plant sources (i.e.: an anti-inflammatory diet). So what's the truth?

The truth is that muscle loss is something that can and does occur with any rapid weight loss. Your body can only metabolize about a pound of fat a week. If your diet is restrictive enough to cause massive weight loss, you can be sure that some of that is muscle. That is why it is suggested to keep calorie restriction to 500 calories below what is needed for maintenance to allow for slow and steady progress and maximum muscle retention. So, what do the studies show?

One study concluded that intermittent fasting gave the same weight loss results as following a calorie-restricted diet. Still, those practicing intermittent fasting had lost less muscle mass than those doing calorie restriction (Varady, 2011). A second study indicated that individuals who consumed one meal a day, taking in their daily calories in one sitting, could proudly flex their muscles as they actually showed an increase in muscle mass (Stote et al., 2007). If done right, you can use your body processes to burn fat for fuel and preserve your muscle mass. Intermittent fasting is the way to do this.

Your Health Is in Jeopardy

This has been one of the most frustrating arguments, as it usually comes from some of the most unhealthy people I know. After my initial weight loss from switching to IF and a plant-based diet, someone close to me said, "You're too skinny." Mind you, I was smack in the middle of the "healthy" BMI range, but I had suddenly dropped under the societal norm. Most of us don't fall into that healthy range anymore. So this person, at more than 100 pounds overweight (from dietary and not health factors), judged me as unhealthy. That belief allowed him to avoid making changes himself.

I can honestly say that both my physical and mental health are better than they have ever been. Study after study has shown that intermittent fasting helps people overcome the health barriers of high blood pressure, obesity, diabetes, asthma, rheumatoid arthritis, and more (Longo & Mattson, 2014). Fasting has withstood the test of time and has proven itself to be neither a "fad" nor a "craze." We will explore the myriad of health benefits in future chapters. Stay with me!

It's All About Your Metabolism

Another common misconception is that IF will shut down your metabolism. Trainers and weight-loss experts tell their clients that they need to eat six to eight small meals daily to boost their metabolism, burn calories, and melt away fat. Do this, don't do that. Eat this, don't eat that. The rules are endless. Truth, please?

A study conducted in 1997, before intermittent fasting became a household name, determined that there was no evidence of the relationship between how many calories are burned and how many times a day you eat (Bellisle et al., 1997). Another study in The American Journal of Clinical Nutrition studied the metabolic rate of 16 individuals participating in intermittent fasting over a three-week time period. The research concluded that individuals lost weight and their metabolic rates were unaffected (Heilbronn et al., 2005).

It is important to note that it is possible to damage your metabolism when dieting. This comes from a severe restriction of calories that triggers your body to go into starvation mode and hold onto its remaining fat stores for future use. This is not, however, a hallmark or consequence of intermittent fasting when done correctly.

You Absolutely Cannot Exercise While Doing IF

I would love to wager a bet that this is more a hope than an actual misconception. It is no secret that exercising is an activity that many people love to hate. I have met many individuals who have told me they don't like going to the gym because of their insecurities. I get that; I honestly do. Thanks to the global pandemic, fitness routines have become more accessible, and we no longer have to go out and exercise in a group or a room full of sweaty bodies.

Can you exercise while following the intermittent fasting lifestyle? Oh, you know what I am going to say—ABSOLUTELY! I'm not going to force you to go to the gym. Still, I am going to encourage you to either take advantage of one of the many online fitness classes or videos or use your home as a fitness studio by using what you already have in your pantry or cleaning closet. Your pantry holds bags or containers filled with flour, rice, or sugar (really best not to eat this, anyway!) which you could use as weights or grab a couple of cans of beans or soup to work on the arm curls. Your cleaning closet houses a broom and a mop that you could bring out of retirement to give your home a good clean and yourself a vigorous cardio workout. The options for exercise are endless—only limited by your imagination!

Is it safe to exercise while following the intermittent fasting lifestyle? The short answer is yes, but you need to listen to your body. No one else knows your body better than you do, so look and listen for signs, and if needed, keep it light. If you are new to exercise, check with your healthcare provider before starting a new routine. The topic of exercise will be continued in Chapter 7, so be sure to stick around.

All Intermittent Fasting Plans Are Created Equal

I've heard it said that comparison is the thief of joy. That can be especially true on a health journey. It is impossible to compare our path or progress with someone else's. Our bodies are each created entirely unique, and things such as muscle mass, bone structure, hormone balance, metabolism, and body fat vary from person to person. Our IF and eating plans need to be just as unique to fit our needs. In Chapter 4, I will go into more detail and discuss various options that you may want to adopt as part of your IF lifestyle.

And the List Goes On...

The myths and misconceptions surrounding intermittent fasting already discussed in this chapter are just the tip of the iceberg. Be prepared to hear more as you start this journey, but remember that the truth is the truth. Don't let the lies and the misconceptions fuel doubt or derail you. Here are a few more, but be assured that you'll hear the truth about these as you continue to read.

- Science and research do not support intermittent fasting.
- Fasting throws your body into starvation mode.
- Breakfast is the most important meal of the day.
- Skipping breakfast will make you gain weight.
- You will overeat when you break your fast.
- It is difficult to concentrate on your work or tasks while fasting.

- Your energy reserves are depleted while fasting.
- Fasting raises your stress levels and affects your moods.
- Fasting deprives your brain of the necessary dietary supply of glucose.
- You are depriving your body of necessary nutrients when eating only one or two meals a day.
- There is no limit to how much you can eat when breaking your fast.

We've heard from the naysayers and the skeptics. We have listened to their criticisms. We can't change how they think, but we can share our own positive experiences and successes with intermittent fasting, to become ambassadors for a healthier way of life. By doing this, we can help pave the way for others to join us. Let's move from the darkness into the light and look at what intermittent fasting really *is* and what it does.

3

INTERMITTENT FASTING IN A NUTSHELL

N ow that we've covered who shouldn't undertake intermittent fasting and what it's not, let's move on to the good stuff. Exactly who can do it, and what is it?

Intermittent fasting has become one of the most popular lifestyles in recent years. In 2020, The International Food Information Council (ICIF) interviewed more than 1,000 individuals about their eating habits. The survey found that approximately 10% of the over 1,000 individuals responding put intermittent fasting in the top spot behind clean eating and the ketogenic diet as their eating pattern of choice. Its popularity is likely attributed to the fact that with IF, there is no product to purchase nor a specific diet to follow. It allows people to make decisions based on their individual needs (Crawford, 2020).

Article after article puts intermittent fasting in the top 10 most popular diets. A quick Google search on "intermittent fasting" will generate a return of over 61,200,000 results. Research has indicated that it has remained a popular life-style choice for years. Are you ready to find out why? If you've been sitting on the fence, now is the time to jump off and follow me as we take an in-depth look at what intermittent fasting is and what it entails.

UNDERSTANDING INTERMITTENT FASTING

Intermittent fasting is an easy concept that can be difficult to grasp if you get bogged down in the plethora of information on the internet. The fact that it is so easy to individualize means that the methods of fasting vary as much as the people practicing it. You'll hear about macros, timing, clean versus dirty, and more. That can get overwhelming. My goal is to cut through the confusion and get down to basics. Let's slow down, take a deep breath, and start at the beginning. I want to show you how easy it is to apply intermittent fasting to your lifestyle. Remember, we all already practice intermittent fasting for a minimum of 6 to 8 hours a night (or day) while sleeping!

The Layman's Definition of Intermittent Fasting

The intermittent fasting lifestyle is designed in such a way as to limit your consumption of calorie-dense food and beverages between certain hours of the day or week. The recommendation from veteran fasters is to focus on your fast lasting anywhere from 12 to 40 hours. I realize that 40 hours sounds daunting, but you don't need to start there, even if you intend to end there. There are many different types of IF programs that you can adopt and apply to your lifestyle—which we will discuss in more detail in Chapter 4.

Intermittent fasting is often referred to as "time-restricted feeding," implying that individuals have a window of opportunity each day to consume their meals.

It's not about what you are going to eat (just yet, but we'll get there) when you break your fast, but it is about the timing. IF doesn't give you a specific list of things to eat—that is up to you! Instead, it tells you when to eat them. This is good news for those who want a way to lose weight and improve their health without changing the foods they eat or increasing their exercise! It is possible to do one without the other. That is one of the things that I love about intermittent fasting—nothing is off-limits. It allows for intuitive eating and stops the obsession with food and thinking about things you can't have. People often find, though, that when they adopt the IF lifestyle, it improves their relationship with food, and they make healthier choices. In that way, intermittent fasting is not a diet but an addition to a controlled eating plan.

I want to assure you that you won't be starving or depriving yourself of food and nutrients. You're effectively learning how to discipline your mind and body into avoiding calorie-dense pastries, donuts, cookies, sodas, and all the foods you might otherwise eat if you weren't on the plan. You will automatically cut back on calories because you are eating for fewer hours in a day—and your food choices will usually improve as you aim to nourish your body as much as possible in that shorter period. Once you get in the nutrients you need, there just isn't time to eat all the junk! It is incredible the number of calories that most of us will cut out when doing away with late-night "grazing" or eating out of boredom. As you transition into this way of eating, your body becomes accustomed to eating smaller portions, including healthier foods and fewer snacks, and the cravings will decrease. No two people are the same, and you will need to find a way of fasting and eating that works for you, but I have heard story after story from people in my online IF groups that said their diet became healthier the longer they practiced IF, even without making a conscious switch.

Intermittent fasting is about making a conscious choice to skip meals so that you only consume your allotted daily calories within the window of your eating cycle. The bonus is that you'll see that fat melt away in the process! It is important to state that because of the inherent calorie reduction, IF shouldn't be undertaken by people who are underweight. You need to have a fat store that can be used to burn for energy in place of glucose.

IT'S ALL GOOD! A LOOK AT THE BENEFITS OF INTERMITTENT FASTING

Now for the good stuff! What do you stand to gain from adopting an intermittent fasting lifestyle? The immediate thought is usually weight loss, and this is often true. But regardless of whether weight loss is one of your goals, IF offers much more. Let's see.

Intermittent Fasting Offers You More Than Weight Loss Solutions—But That IS a Benefit!

I think it's safe to assume you know that weight loss and maintenance are some of the biggest benefits of intermittent fasting. For many of us over 50, that's exactly what we're seeking. Changes in lifestyle and hormones over the years make it harder for most women to achieve and maintain a healthy weight. Intermittent fasting can definitely help with that. Millions of people have found success with IF, whereas other diets have failed them. Some of us have stubborn weight to lose, and IF can help with that as well. When your body switches to fat-burning for fuel (discussed later), it reduces areas often untouched by other diets—like the dreaded belly fat! That is what I discovered when I switched to IF nearly four years ago. I broke through a weight plateau that I had previously been sitting on for more than 15 years. When done in conjunction with an optimal diet, IF can help you gradually attain and maintain a healthy weight. Good weight loss solutions (like IF) are not focused on losing the most weight in the shortest amount of time but are about losing weight slowly and steadily, so you don't risk undoing all your hard work and damaging your health in the process.

Control over your eating is paramount for weight loss to occur with IF. Especially in the beginning, before your body has become accustomed to the prolonged period of fasting, you may be tempted to shove anything and everything into your mouth once your fast has ended. Like, immediately after. Developing a strategy to combat this is important. Donate high-calorie snacks to a homeless shelter for women and children. Stock your fridge and pantry with low-calorie fresh fruit, veggies, nuts, seeds, hummus, soups, and other quick-to-grab meals and snacks. Listen to your body. Eat slowly. Do not deprive yourself—instead, eat when you're hungry and stop when you're full. Practice intuitive eating. Listen to your body because your mind will play hardball in the beginning and try to derail you, but it will catch up when it realizes that you are serious about your new lifestyle.

While the overall focus of IF should be health improvement and not weight loss, it is important to take note of your weight during your intermittent fasting journey. You want to maintain a healthy weight. First, you want your weight loss, if any, to be slow and steady. A pound a week is optimal. If you find that you are losing too rapidly or dropping below what is recommended for your height and age, gradually increase your calorie intake so that you don't undo all the work you have already done. Believe it or not, it is also possible to gain weight when you first begin doing IF. This is especially true if you are subscribing to the "eat whatever you want during your eating window" philosophy. Weighing yourself can identify an over-indulgence in calories and quickly get you back on track. I also want to acknowledge that some of us (myself included) suffer from health conditions that will not allow us to lose all of our unwanted pounds, no matter how hard we try. Intermittent fasting is for us, too, because, as you will see next, it is more about health and added benefits than weight loss. We, too, can fall in love with our bodies again, and that is the ultimate goal. Let's look at some other health benefits we can look forward to.

Autophagy

Intermittent fasting is beneficial to the body because it helps your body enter a state of autophagy. This process assists your body with repairing and repurposing cells that have been damaged or have become redundant. Your body is a virtual industrial plant of organs, tissues, cells, and muscles, as well as an intricate web of veins that are working overtime to ensure that everything inside you works like a well-oiled machine. Despite our best efforts, as we age, the parts start malfunctioning. This can be a wake-up call that it's time to make some much-needed alterations to our current lifestyle.

When the body enters the state of fasting and autophagy kicks in, it starts sorting through our cells, separates the good, bad, and damaged cells, and sends them off for quality control. Those cells are either repaired, recycled, or discarded. Autophagy allows the body to repurpose our cells, thus rejuvenating our bodies. While autophagy is continually happening in our bodies, intermittent fasting stimulates the process and helps us maximize it for optimum health and energy. In addition, autophagy can decrease our body fat percentage (Cleveland Clinic, n.d.). Autophagy for the win!

Better Cardiovascular Health

Intermittent fasting shows promise in improving several aspects of cardiovascular health. Though more research is needed to determine all the mechanisms behind this, it is believed that many come from the benefits of weight loss and decreased body fat. Intermittent fasting has been attributed to lower metabolic energy consumption, lower blood pressure, decreased low-density cholesterol levels, including triglycerides, reduction in sleep apnea, improved oxygen dispersion in the body, and decreased insulin resistance, which can improve or eliminate Type II diabetes. Intermittent fasting has been attributed to increased longevity, and an improvement in cardiovascular health is undoubtedly one of the factors contributing to this. (Varady et al., 2021).

Reduced Inflammation

Everyone has inflammation. It is a natural body process that assists in fighting infections, harmful bacteria, and whatever your body considers a foreign entity. Once your immune system detects these dangers, it alerts your body's cellular army (inflammation), and the battle for healing begins. When your body loses this battle, it can lead to chronic inflammation, which wreaks havoc by attacking muscles, cells, or tissues and can cause a host of other diseases and disorders. (Pahwa & Jialal, 2019).

Intermittent fasting to the rescue! In 2012, researchers studied a group of patients diagnosed with chronic and acute cases of inflammation. When following a calorie-restricted diet, there was a reduction in inflammation levels as well as the proinflammatory cytokines circulating in the blood. Even better, their life expectancy was extended. (Faris et al., 2012).

Improved Brain Function

When you think of brain health, you may not immediately think of diet. The truth is that what you eat and how you eat it greatly impacts your mental functioning. The standard American diet (SAD), with its high intake of refined carbohydrates, sugar, and fat, has been linked to not only emotional and mood disorders but also cognitive impairment in both human and animal studies. When paired with a nutritious diet, intermittent fasting has instead been shown to be extremely beneficial in improving brain health and cognitive function. It can ease brain fog and enhance memory. In extreme cases, IF can even counteract or prevent disorders such as Parkinson's and Alzheimer's, dementia, seizure disorder, and multiple sclerosis. (Gudden et al., 2021).

Decreased Leptin Resistance

One of the biggest benefits of IF is that it encourages weight loss because your brain is blocked from identifying hunger pangs. This mental block prevents your mind from telling you that you're hungry. This effect is the work of the satiety hormone, otherwise known as leptin. Many of us suffer from leptin resistance and are unable to recognize when we are full. As a result, we are constantly hungry. That is where intermittent fasting comes into play.

IF decreases inflammation that causes leptin resistance and resets the leptin receptors, allowing them to work properly again. This will increase your satisfaction when eating and decrease food cravings. Together, these factors will decrease your overall calorie intake and allow for greater weight loss when fasting. Our stomachs make another hormone called ghrelin, which is an appetite stimulant. It encourages eating, and studies have shown that increased ghrelin is found in many people with eating disorders. Increased leptin levels help to decrease ghrelin, further aiding in our eating control. Following the IF lifestyle will help you reduce the ghrelin hormones and can also increase the "happy hormone" dopamine in your brain (Kucine, 2018). Wins all around!

Why Does Intermittent Fasting Work?

The majority of testing on IF has been done on animal models, so it is a bit early in its history to say definitively why it works, especially on humans. What we do know is this, in terms of weight loss:

- Intermittent fasting limits the number of meals a person eats in a day and will also generally decrease the number of calories they are consuming.
- Not eating for 10–16 hours triggers your body to burn its fat stores for energy. This may not only result in extra fat loss but also account for people who lose weight on IF despite no calorie reduction.
- Improvement in "eating hormones" will increase your satiation and decrease your overall feelings of hunger and cravings.

In terms of health benefits and disease reduction:

- Ketones are released into the bloodstream once your body starts burning fat for energy. They improve memory, learning processes, and also slow various disease processes in the brain (Mattson, 2011).
- The calorie reduction from IF (i.e., "undernutrition without malnutrition") is likely the key component in slowing cancer growth (Freedland et al., 2010).
- Fasting for periods of 16 or more hours decreases insulin levels. This is not only helpful for weight loss

but is also key to lowering the risk of various diseases, including but not limited to diabetes and pre-diabetes (Miller, 2022).

It is not within the scope of this book to go into great detail regarding the physiology behind intermittent fasting and how it affects each of the body's processes. A few other authors have undertaken this, and I will refer you to their books. I desire to bring you a practical guide that is easy to read, easy to use, and can give you the tools to start your fasting journey soon. However, it is important to understand at least the basics, which are this—intermittent fasting addresses both weight and health primarily through two mechanisms: calorie reduction during the eating window and the process changes in the body during the fasting period. Some of those processes have been addressed above, and we will look at more in future chapters.

Potential Negative Effects of Intermittent Fasting

I would love to tell you that intermittent fasting has no downsides. Wouldn't that be amazing? Unfortunately, though IF is an excellent way to improve health and lose weight, it isn't a magic bullet. The good news is that most of the adverse effects of IF will resolve or can be avoided if done correctly. As I've said before, intermittent fasting is a lifestyle that you will perfect through trial and error, as there is no one-size-fits-all plan. As your body adapts to the changes it is going through, you should come out the other side victorious. So let's take a look at what you might experience.

- **Intense hunger and cravings**: The early days of transitioning may be challenging, but feelings of intense hunger or cravings should decrease and even be eliminated eventually. Perseverance is the key!
- **Dehydration**: You are reminded to keep an eye on the color of your urine as IF typically flushes your body of salts and toxins. Remember to drink lots of water and non-caloric beverages during your fasting window to keep your kidneys happy.
- **Labile moods**: Social media created a word for the lack of food and the attitude that goes with it— "hangry"—and you may experience this in the beginning. Eventually, your body will adapt, and you will be your sweet self again.
- **Intermittent fasting breath**: You may have heard the term "keto breath," and this is the same. It is an unpleasant taste in the mouth and bad breath caused by ketosis (your body burning your fat storage), and your body releasing the toxins and chemicals from that process through your exhalation. This usually lasts from a few days to a couple of weeks and will subside once your body adapts.
- **Digestive issues**: The negative effects may include a change in the frequency of passing stools, nausea, bloating, or diarrhea. This can also be attributed to

the increase in fiber when switching to a more plant-strong diet. Again, this will adapt once your body adjusts to your new eating pattern.

- **Headaches**: The headaches and the feeling of moving with your head in the clouds will settle down as you adapt to IF—consume lots of water and only do light exercise until you have adapted.

- **Weakness and fatigue**: This can be caused by either a lack of sufficient calories to meet your daily needs or electrolyte imbalances. Try adding a pinch of sea salt to your morning coffee or water. You may need to track calories, in the beginning, to ensure you have a good idea of your needs, consumption, and expenditure.

- **Insomnia**: In early phases, IF may affect your sleeping patterns—either not being able to fall asleep or struggling to stay asleep because your body is adjusting to the changes (Kubala, 2021). This too shall pass.

- **Medication effects**: I have previously mentioned that it is crucial to consult your healthcare provider before undertaking IF or any other change in your current lifestyle. Because of the changes taking place in your body, your current medications may affect you differently and need to be monitored or adjusted as you progress. Remember, the goal of this lifestyle is not to put your health at risk but rather to help you find the perfect balance (Frey, 2020).

MY INTRODUCTION TO INTERMITTENT FASTING

I was all over the place the first time I tried intermittent fasting! I didn't really know the whys or hows behind how it worked or how to do it. I had just heard a zillion stories of people able to eat anything they wanted and still lose weight. That was my dream! I had spent my whole life depriving myself of food, yet I was overweight. I had tried every craze and fad diet out there, and nothing worked. This sounded too good to be true. Well, of course, in a way, it was. My first attempt included starving myself for as long as I could during the day and then bingeing uncontrollably on unhealthy processed foods during my eating window. I was so hungry by the time I was allowed to eat that I ate anything and everything in sight. I am guessing that I had effectively doubled the number of daily calories that I normally ate because of my insatiable hunger.

I tried adopting a shorter fasting window and lengthening my eating window. I didn't pay much attention to how this corresponded with my usual eating patterns, though, and it turns out that I wasn't experiencing much of a fast beyond what I normally did. I was allowed to eat for a full 8-hour window each day. I was still buying into the "eat anything you want" mentality, and the result was that I was back to my old eating pattern in regard to timing, but I was increasing my calorie intake due to my no-boundaries approach to what I was putting in my mouth. Not surprisingly, no weight loss for me. I yo-yoed back and forth between IF experiments, but with much the same results. I was tired. I had headaches. My mood was awful. Instead of finding freedom from obsessing about food, I was constantly thinking about it. Even worse, I wasn't losing weight. Instead, I felt like I was losing ground.

That was when I began to realize that there is science behind IF and which method to choose needs to be carefully considered. This isn't a one-size-fits-all lifestyle, just like we aren't one-size-fits-all people. I learned that IF is most effective if you focus on health and not weight. If you do that, the weight will usually follow. In the coming chapters, we will discuss all of this in more detail and get you on the right path.

4

10 TYPES OF INTERMITTENT FASTING—PICKING YOUR WINNER!

This chapter will explore 10 types of intermittent fasting lifestyle programs. I will guide you through each program and give you all the information in a clear, concise, and easy-to-understand format. The program you choose to follow should be the one that best suits your lifestyle, so make sure to examine each one carefully.

Intermittent fasting is one of the most popular weight loss approaches among Americans, and its popularity is growing worldwide. I have spoken to people from all over who have shared their IF journeys with me. Studies indicate that 24% of people in the US have tried IF for weight loss, and it is tied in popularity with the Atkins diet, Weight Watchers, and Keto. The great thing about intermittent fasting is that it can be used in conjunction with any healthy eating plan because IF is not a diet. Nine out of ten people who have previously tried IF reported that it was either very effective or at least moderately effective in helping them lose weight.

I have heard many people talk about the cost of following a healthy eating plan or how much money they have to spend on supplements and shakes. The truth is that IF doesn't have to break the bank! Based on a recent poll, 80% of individuals who participated in intermittent fasting found it inexpensive, while only 18% found it more expensive than their previous eating habits (Ballard, 2020). I'd say that the statistics speak for themselves.

TYPES OF INTERMITTENT FASTING

This is the moment we've all been waiting for—a walk-through of the various types of intermittent fasting plans. Each section will feature important information, including the pros and cons of each method. My goal is for you to have everything you need to make an informed decision about the direction in which you want to steer your IF journey.

Daily Time-Restricted Fasting

Time-restricted fasting allows you to eat normally BUT only within a set window of hours. Contrary to what you may think, many people experience less hunger during their fast when they do a longer fasting window and a shorter eating window than when they do a shorter fasting window and a longer eating window. The longer fasting times can decrease hunger signals as well as cravings (remember our friend leptin?). It is, however, important to note that there has yet to be a definitive consensus on when the process of autophagy begins in the body during fasting. Some studies have shown autophagy to start within as little as 12 hours of fasting, while others believe it does not begin until somewhere between 24–48 hours.

16:8

With this method, you will be fasting for 16 hours and eating during an 8-hour window. Thus, 16:8 is one of the most popular time-restricted fasting plans. It allows for maximum flexibility and minimum disruption to your eating habits and lifestyle and still provides immeasurable health benefits. Studies have shown improvements in blood sugar control, weight loss, and longevity in subjects adhering to a 16:8 window. This can be done for as little or as frequently as you'd like, such as once or twice a week or even daily. However, it is important to let you know that the benefits will be maximized and more noticeable the more often you do it. The most common eating windows for people on a 16:8 schedule are:

- 9 a.m. to 5 p.m.
- 10 a.m. to 6 p.m.
- 12 p.m. to 8 p.m.

You will need to experiment with the schedule to see what works best for you and your lifestyle. The 16:8 is a good place for those just starting IF. The extended eating window may be a potential downside, however, for people needing to lose weight. It gives you more time to consume an abundance of calories, thus possibly not promoting weight loss. Eating within a 16:8 schedule requires intentionality.

18:6

This is another popular form of intermittent fasting. It potentially yields more significant weight loss than the 16:8 method. By following this specific schedule, individuals abstain from consuming food for a period of 18 hours and then have a six-hour window in which to consume their meals. It is a bit more intense than 16:8, so you may want to start with a shorter fasting window and work your way up to the 18-hour fast.

One of the most important benefits of the 18:6 fasting schedule may include a good night's rest—providing the eating window doesn't end too close to bedtime. Other benefits include improved gut health, decreased bloating due to adequate time for digestion of food, proper rest for the GI system, reduced insulin resistance, decreased brain fog and other cognitive benefits, heightened energy levels, and lower inflammation. Another marked benefit of the 18:6 plan is that you can eat larger meals in one sitting, increasing satisfaction over eating multiple smaller meals throughout the day. And yes, that is excellent news for those of us that like to eat!

The downside to the 18:6 schedule is that you may be left feeling restricted because your meals must fall within a small window, and you may experience intense hunger during your fasting periods (especially if you are not consuming adequate calories or nutrients during the eating window). This could be a trigger for binge eating or open the door to other eating disorders.

20:4

The benefits of a 20:4 window include:

- **Improved body composition**: 20:4 puts your body in a state of increased beta-oxidation, and your liver begins to produce ketones, both of which result in burning fat stores for fuel.
- **Improved insulin sensitivity**: The state of ketosis will also boost your body's insulin sensitivity; food consumption will result in muscle growth rather than glucose production.
- **Improved cellular health**: Twenty hours of fasting should see your body solidify in autophagy, which is the process wherein your body heals and repairs itself. During the fasting period, stem cell production —which undoes the effects of cellular wear-and-tear and provides the body with youthful energy —skyrockets.

- **Increased HGH production**: Human growth hormone production increases, contributing to improved muscle mass, better memory, reduced water retention, and decreased cortisol (stress hormone) levels.
- **Increased brain-derived neurotrophic factor (BDNF)**: Your BDNF is responsible for increased brain cell production, faster learning, and neural pathway development. High levels of BDNF protect against degenerative neuro disorders such as Alzheimer's and Parkinson's diseases.
- **Reduced inflammation**: In addition to "normal" inflammation, 20 hours of fasting can also help counteract inflammation in the GI tract, known as the "leaky gut syndrome." This syndrome is associated with food allergies, inflammatory disorders, and autoimmune disorders such as MS, Sjogren's, and rheumatoid arthritis (McAuliffe, 2022).
- **Improved productivity**: On a less scientific front, IF can lead to improvement in overall daily productivity as you spend much less time shopping for food, as well as preparing, eating, and cleaning up after meals—this can translate into financial savings as well!

The 20:4 fasting schedule is a very intense regimen. Even though the fasting window is only two hours longer than

18:6, individuals may experience intense hunger during the fasting period. It may lead to hormonal disruption in women, leading to irregular menstrual cycles, ovary size, and decreased bone density for women over 50. Hormone disruptions could increase food cravings, leading to less satiety after eating, which can trigger binge eating and eating disorders in some women.

Benefits of Time-Restricted Fasting

One of the main benefits of time-restricted fasting is that limiting the number of hours you eat each day, combined with a healthy diet, may help you naturally consume fewer calories. The fewer calories you consume over a period of time, the more likely you are to obtain and maintain optimal weight. Scientists have conducted time-restricted fasting studies on both animal and human subjects, and results showed the additional benefits of an increased lifespan in rats and decreased inflammation in humans (Alhamdan et al., 2016).

Another article found that individuals who practice short-term IF have an increase in metabolism of up to 14%. The belief is that during short-term IF, the stress hormone that is the gatekeeper for the fatty acids—norepinephrine—rises and releases larger fatty deposits into the bloodstream for the body to recycle. When your metabolic rate increases because of short-term intermittent fasting, you will burn calories when you sleep, relax, or even enjoy dinner. It must also be mentioned that exercise is encouraged to help build muscle (Mehmet, 2021).

Many new converts to the intermittent fasting lifestyle have shared that the time restriction doesn't faze them, as they still maintain their normal eating habits. They have indicated that they still eat the foods they enjoy and continue to lose weight and burn excess fat. Intermittent fasting doesn't control your life. You get to build your time restriction around your schedule, which allows for flexibility—especially when you are out socializing because you can consume whatever your friends are eating during your specific time period. Always remember that YOU are in charge of your IF journey, which means you can plan your fasting and eating windows schedule to fit into your lifestyle. The most crucial factor that you need to remember is that you reap the benefits of fasting by consuming your meals only during your eating window. The longer you can fast, the fewer calories you will likely consume. You are then more likely to kick your body into autophagy, and you will reap the fruits of your fasting.

One study of 90 participants conducted in Pakistan showed increased benefits to keeping your eating window early in the day. They found that, compared with normal eating over a period of 12 or more hours, time-restricted eating starting earlier in the day was more effective for mood regulation, weight loss, and diastolic blood pressure reduction (Bascom, 2022).

Remember that we have discussed the potential dangers of adopting the fasting lifestyle if suffering from disordered eating, but there are also potential benefits. It is widely speculated that fasting may help improve your relationship with food. As eating during your fasting window is not an option, you will learn to find alternative ways to cope with your stress, boredom, labile emotions, or any other reasons that lead you to overeat. Fasting may also be seen as an aid to assist you in replacing your food addictions with various other coping mechanisms—especially when you practice mindfulness when eating. Creating a food and fasting journal may help (more on that soon).

The 5:2 Method

As previously mentioned in Chapter 2, Dr. Michael Mosley popularized intermittent fasting when he wrote, produced, and presented a documentary for BBC, as well as wrote various books about the IF lifestyle. He is the founder of the 5:2 method, where you eat according to your usual habits five days a week and limit your calories to between 500 to 600 for the other two days. It is very important to know your portion sizes when following this method and to weigh and measure your food as accurately as possible to ensure that you stay within the limited caloric window. The five "normal" days are not an open invitation to cram in as much calorie-dense food as you can. It is quite possible to undo the benefits of your two days of fasting if you do not eat healthy food on the other five.

You do not have any set requirements for what you eat while following the 5:2 IF method, except that you cannot (should not) consume more than 600 calories on your two fasting days. You are in control of your schedule, and you can choose any two days of the week to fast. However, you have to ensure that you have at least one non-fasting day in between. Do not fast on two consecutive days. You should also disperse your calories throughout your fasting days so you don't consume everything in one sitting. If at all possible, try to consume the same amount of food on your non-fasting days as you normally would. Should you be prepping for your fasting day by overeating the day before to compensate, you will increase your overall calorie count for the week. This can be a setback that risks you gaining back all the weight and undoing all the positive changes you have already accomplished.

There are no definitive studies on the benefits or effects of the 5:2 fasting method, but with that in mind, I would like to share a couple of potential pros and cons with you.

One of the benefits of the 5:2 fasting method is that all the focus is on your eating schedule. You don't have any limits to the food you consume during your "feasting" days. You may even be more likely to adhere to your schedule knowing that you don't have restrictions. Though it has not been proven, it can be assumed that the confirmed benefits of following the other types of IF would also apply to the 5:2 method.

The downside of this IF method is that individuals may experience severe hunger on fasting days. Hunger can lead you to inadvertently consume more than your allotted 500- to 600-calorie limit or break the fast altogether. Other potential downsides are that individuals may experience weakness, exhaustion, or brain fog because of the low caloric intake on fasting days.

Alternate Day Fasting (ADF)

This intermittent fasting method is where you limit or refrain from food every other day and eat normally on the days you are not fasting. You may find purists who will only consume water, herbal tea, or moderate amounts of black coffee (no sugar) on fasting days; others may adopt the 25% rule. This rule states that you may consume 25% of your normal calories (500 to 600) on your fasting days. The ADF is similar to the 5:2 method, but as the name implies, you fast on alternate days. Instead of the 5:2 method, you end up with the equivalent of a 4:3 schedule. It is vitally important to remain hydrated by consuming non-caloric and unsweetened beverages on fasting days.

This is considered one of the more extreme versions of the intermittent fasting lifestyle, and many individuals find it difficult to follow in the long term. You may find it more beneficial to follow this method occasionally when you want to "reset" the neurons in your brain that control the hunger signals and overeating triggers. Studies have proven that the

ADF is more sustainable when allowing 500 calories on fasting days than if not consuming anything at all. One study played two of the fasting methods up against each other— ADF and time-restricted. The drop-out rate for the ADF study was 30% of their subjects, and the time-restricted group had little to no drop-outs (Millard, 2020).

Like the other less-common methods of IF, few, if any, studies have been done on the pros and cons of ADF specifically. It is worthwhile to mention, though, that many sources issue warnings against women practicing the ADF method because it may potentially disrupt female hormone levels. One small study involving women following the alternate-day fasting method for three weeks noted that they had worse blood sugar control than before adopting the fasting lifestyle (Heilbronn, Civitarese, et al., 2005).

The 36-Hour Fast

The 36-hour fast, also called the "Monk Fast," is an advanced version of intermittent fasting that typically requires individuals to skip one entire day of eating. The principle of the 36-hour fast is that individuals finish their dinner at 7:30 p.m. on day one and then skip food on day two. They are then advised to break their fast at 7:30 a.m. on day three. You can choose your meal times, but the stopping time on day one has to coincide with the morning eating time on day three. A fasting expert and physician, Dr. Jason Fung, recommends that patients to his clinic participate in three 36-hour fasts a week to help them with their type 2 diabetes. It is highly recommended that this type of intense fasting should only be undertaken with full physician supervision.

As previously mentioned, the 36-hour fast is advanced and extreme, and individuals new to the IF journey may find it difficult. One of the downsides to this type of IF plan is the possibility of becoming hypoglycemic, where blood sugar levels become too low for the body to function properly. This is of particular concern for people with poor blood sugar regulation (Warren, 2022).

The 24-Hour Fast (or Eat-Stop-Eat)

The 24-hour fast works on the same principle as the 5:2 method, but you can choose whether to fast on one or two (non-consecutive) days a week—depending on your goals. The fasting times are up to you, but once you stop eating, you will not have your next meal for a full 24 hours. You are encouraged to have a meal before your fast commences. Remember to remain hydrated throughout your 24-hour fast by drinking unsweetened non-caloric beverages.

As we've seen previously, the pros and cons of each of these plans are similar. Like the others, the 24-hour fast potentially supports weight loss, speeds up metabolism, improves blood pressure and blood sugar levels, and simplifies food options. The potential downsides are also the same—irritability, mood changes, hunger, fatigue, and hormone disruptions. For this reason, these types of intense IF schedules should not be undertaken by pregnant women, children, or those with chronic health conditions without supervision by a medical care provider (Hill, 2022).

One Meal A Day (OMAD)

As the name of this fasting plan suggests, you consume one meal a day. You do not consume any other calories outside of that one meal. The fasting and eating window for OMAD plans is typically 23:1, where you consume all your calories within one hour. Most individuals opt to consume their meals in the evening. It is believed that the ideal time to break the fast is anywhere between 4 p.m. to 7 p.m. each day. This is the time most people spend time with family or friends, and it allows you to refuel your energy and ensures that you give your food adequate time to digest before going to bed. There are no conclusive studies to support or refute the benefits or downsides of consuming your meals upon waking or in the late afternoon or evening.

If you want to adopt the OMAD fasting plan, it is ideally advised to start with a less restrictive type of intermittent fasting and build up from there. If you are a beginner, you should start by fasting between 16 and 20 hours. As you get used to the effects, you can work up to OMAD gradually until you are comfortable and confident enough to do it daily. I know many people following OMAD who have adopted a "no holds barred" approach to their mealtime. They eat anything and everything they want within their one-hour window. This is a benefit for some—they can focus on their timeframe for eating and not be bothered with what they consume. That said, the best results I have seen have been achieved by those who also focus on clean eating to ensure that they are fueling their body adequately.

Some of the benefits of following the OMAD fasting plan are as follows:

- rapid weight loss
- easy to follow
- no need to count calories
- no food is off limits
- meal preparation is simple and reduces time spent focusing on meals
- inexpensive lifestyle plan
- slows down aging
- boosts your metabolic health
- prolongs autophagy (fat loss and body healing)

The downsides to the OMAD fasting plan are varied and controversial, and more research is called for. Though you are almost guaranteed to show weight loss results, some individuals do experience problems which include the following:

- increased body fat percentage
- increased cholesterol levels
- increased blood pressure

- risk of binge eating and triggering eating disorders
- difficulty in adhering to the strict fasting schedule
- feelings of weakness, exhaustion, irritability, and trouble concentrating
- not being flexible to allow for socializing with friends outside of your window of eating
- difficulty in consuming adequate calories in one sitting which could cause muscle wasting, malnutrition, or a slower metabolism
- disruption of reproductive hormones

The Warrior Diet

The Warrior Diet was developed by Ori Hofmekler in 2001. This method is based on the beliefs of the creator and not science. The Warrior Diet falls under the umbrella of the intermittent fasting lifestyle but has a few modifications. The basic principle of this diet is that individuals follow in the footsteps of ancient warriors who "grazed" during the day and "feasted" at night.

The creator had a vision in mind when he developed this diet, which was designed to improve the way you perform, the way you look, and the way you eat. The bottom line is to stress the body by limiting the amount of food being consumed and preparing it for survival mode. This method does not prevent you from eating outside of your eating window, but it does encourage individuals to consume as little as possible for 20 hours and enjoy an unlimited feast during the following four hours.

The 20-hour "fasting" period allows you to consume dairy, eggs, fruits, and vegetables in small quantities throughout the day. Remember to consume as many non-caloric beverages as possible to prevent dehydration. Individuals who follow this method have reported that their concentration has improved, they have more energy, and they are burning fat. It is important to note that this is a very controversial plan with no science to back it. This way of eating is similar to the "dirty fast," which I will introduce you to in the next section.

Clean Versus Dirty

Clean fasting is when you follow one of the intermittent fasting protocols and only consume unsweetened non-caloric beverages, which include tap, mineral, and sparkling water, as well as black teas and coffee during your fast. Any beverages with a sweet flavor or taste like food—regardless of the calorie content—are not allowed. These beverages may trigger your body to release insulin to prepare for the calories that are to follow. That means that your body will be kicked out of fasting mode. You may still enjoy the benefits of reduced calories during your fast, but you will potentially stop the fasting process and the benefits that come with it, like autophagy, fat burning, and a boost in your metabolism. Have lots of water but remember that while clean fasting, steer clear of additives like lemon slices and juice, fruit, herbs, and cucumber. While they add flavor to your water, they can also defeat the purpose of a "clean" fast.

Dirty fasting is when you consume food or beverages during your fasting window. This version permits individuals to consume diet drinks, sweeteners, and other additions to tea and coffee that do not exceed the 100-calorie threshold. Your fasting is considered dirty if you add a dash of cream to your tea or coffee, sip on some bone broth, drink zero-calorie soda, or even add zero-calorie sweeteners to your tea or coffee.

There is a lot of controversy surrounding the use of artificial and non-caloric sweeteners used as additives to beverages and whether they contribute to the rise in blood sugar or insulin resistance. Some studies have found no correlation, while others have. One study conducted in 2020 found that the consumption of artificial sweeteners has a negative effect on blood glucose levels. The pancreas is tricked into releasing insulin when individuals consume artificial sweeteners. The sweetness and the similarity to sugar confuse the pancreas, which believes it is glucose. This increases the insulin levels in the blood, which diminishes the activity of receptors due to insulin resistance (Mathur et al., 2020).

It is important to remember that most people who are following the intermittent fasting lifestyle are doing it for health benefits and not just weight loss and management. Non-calorie sweeteners—type dependent—can have potential adverse health effects, and many have been proven to be anything but healthy. Regardless of whether or not they break the fast, it may be best just to steer clear.

I have mentioned multiple times that it is strongly recommended that you stay hydrated throughout your fasting period, and it is worth mentioning again. You are free to drink any unflavored and unsweetened water, tea, or coffee. There is one thing you may add, though—a pinch of pink Himalayan salt to help keep your electrolytes up. All of this liquid can cause a decreased sodium level, which has various effects on how we feel and function. Try this trick if you are feeling lightheaded or struggling with weakness or fatigue.

I have had people ask whether their medication will break their fast, and this is a question best answered by your healthcare provider. Do not ever alter your medication schedule without their consent. Most prescription medication comes with specific directions for being taken with food or on an empty stomach—follow the directions as specified. On a side note, and to ease your mind, most medications will not break your fast unless they are fat-based, sweetened, or high in calories, such as gummies and CBD oil.

Up-to-the-Ninth-Hour Fast

Individuals choosing to adopt this fasting method will abstain from eating for up to eight hours after awaking. Meals are consumed from the ninth hour on. This is rumored to be an ancient form of IF where food is not consumed until 3 p.m. daily. It appears to have its roots in

Christianity, particularly the Catholic faith. It is observed during religious periods such as Lent and is considered a sacrificial act. The fast works on the principle that if your day starts at 6 a.m., you will have your first meal at 3 p.m., which would be the ninth hour. The length of your fasting window would depend on what time you stop eating each day. Research has yet to analyze the up-to-the-ninth-hour fast, but it is widely believed that the pros and cons would be similar to those of other time-restricted fasting methods and dependent on the duration of the time fasted.

Nightly

It is safe to assume that almost every one of us participates in this nightly fast. Eating when you are sleeping is impossible, so you are naturally fasting. This nighttime fasting will last from after your evening meal or bedtime snack until you wake up the following morning. Depending on when we stop eating and what time we wake up in the morning, our nightly fasts are generally 8–12 hours long.

A 2016 study concluded that fasting while sleeping has positive effects on carcinogenesis and the metabolic process. These processes are linked with the risk of breast cancer in women, and fasting decreases that risk. It is believed that a 12-hour fast is generally considered healthy for all individuals. It gives your body a chance to digest the food and beverages consumed and prepare your body for the next day. You also have a decreased risk of being diagnosed with gallstones and gallbladder issues compared to those who fast for longer periods (Marinac et al., 2016).

ONE SIZE DOESN'T FIT ALL

Regardless of the schedule you choose for your intermittent fasting, it is my recommendation that you do a clean fast. If you want to maximize your mental and physical health, you want to stay in the fasting state during your window. My recommendation aside, the best dietary lifestyle is the one that you will stick to. You will have to find what works best for you. Intermittent fasting is not designed to interrupt your busy life; it is meant to conform to your lifestyle.

Choosing the Right Fit

No one can tell you what is going to work for you. The only person who can do that is you. You need to choose an intermittent fasting plan that checks the boxes of who you are, your goals, the flexibility of your eating schedule, or how it will affect your lifestyle. Let's look at a couple of essential questions that you need to ask yourself before making a potentially life-changing decision.

- Do you have a busy social life?
- Do you need a plan that adapts to your socializing commitments?
- Which one of the ten plans grabbed your attention, and why?

- Which one do you believe will fit you and your lifestyle best?
- Do you have health issues that are encouraging you to adopt the IF lifestyle? Or ones that are contraindicated?

The next steps may seem overwhelming, and getting started may seem daunting, but take a deep breath and let's take a look at some practical suggestions. Start with a less restrictive plan. See how that method works for you, and iron out any kinks you may experience. If it's working, either stick with that or progress to a slightly more advanced method. Not seeing the desired results? Try keeping a food and fasting journal where you document the times you fast and what you are consuming (and at what time of the day)—even water. Pay close attention and document anything you put in your mouth. I mean anything. Did you pop a chip in your mouth or lick your greasy, salty fingers when packing lunches for the kids? Maybe you cooked dinner ahead for the family and taste-tested the sauce for saltiness or spice level. A couple of hours before your fasting window arrived, did you reach for a sip of your partner's wine? These things are not the end of the world, but they can add up and push your calories over the edge or contaminate a clean fast. Keeping a journal will allow you to be intentional about what you put into your body and when. But remember—IF is about food freedom. Life happens, and tomorrow is always another day. All is not lost!

Since we are all different, it would be hard to definitively tell why a particular IF method isn't working for you, but there are some common IF mistakes to keep in mind. We've discussed that eating too many calories in your eating window or "off days" can stall weight loss, but eating too few calories can also affect your metabolism by slowing it down. Pay attention to an inadvertent drastic change in calories due to the lifestyle change. If you have paired IF with increased exercise, you may feel excess hunger and then eat more calories in your eating window than you burned during your workout. This is where a journal may come in handy. Dehydration can be another cause of excess feelings of hunger or fatigue, so drink, drink, drink that water. Skipping meals, breaking your fast early, not following the basic guidelines of your method, not sleeping enough, poor food choices, and poor planning are other factors that can derail your efforts. Analyzing your habits carefully can help pinpoint whether your lack of success with IF is related to your own behaviors or if the plan really isn't working for you.

Look at what you can do to make things easier for yourself. Cycle through the IF time-restricted plans until you find one that fits your comfort level. Pick one that you believe will help you realize the goals you have set for yourself. Focus on slow and steady, and remember that the goal should be sustainable good health and not rapid weight loss. Learn to listen to your body, and pay attention to how it feels. Adjust or back off from a plan if you begin to feel consistent adverse effects, or transition to a less intense version of your current method to find a happy medium. Tweak, tweak, and tweak again. That is the key!

MY ONE MEAL-A-DAY EXPERIENCE

I tried OMAD once. That's about all I could handle. I know —you can't try something just once and say that it definitely wasn't a good idea! But trust me... This did NOT feel like a good idea. I like to eat. It was brutal for me to be without eating for 23 hours of my day. Where I should have felt the freedom from thinking about food, I was obsessing about it ALL DAY LONG! By the time my eating window arrived, I was famished. I binge-ate more than my daily needed calories (more than 2,300!) in a one-hour sitting. Ugh.

I made unhealthy choices because I was craving salt, fat, and sugar due to being deprived of calories for 23 hours. What made this whole experience worse was that my meal ended only a few hours before bedtime! I went to bed with a stomach full of about 3,000 calories worth of food. I couldn't sleep, was uncomfortable, and had night sweats all night. I was miserable for days. I had definitely learned my lesson. OMAD is not for everyone.

My message to you is this: Learn from my lesson, too, and start slow. Then work your way up. Don't measure yourself against what others are doing or some lofty goal you've set for yourself. Please don't pick a method you think you should be doing, regardless of whether it's right for you. Instead, set small, reasonable goals and increase your intensity when the time is right. An individualized IF plan is one you'll stick to and reap maximum benefits from. Isn't that really the ultimate goal?

5

WHAT GENDER REVEALS ABOUT WEIGHT LOSS

I have previously mentioned that no two people are the same and that their intermittent fasting journeys will differ due to various contributing factors, including body composition, bone structure, and age. Another key component is gender.

Researchers at the University of New South Wales conducted studies to determine whether there was a link between women storing fat more efficiently than men and the female sex hormone estrogen. The results were conclusive: A woman's body consists of between six and eleven percent more body fat than members of the opposite sex, and estrogen is the culprit. Women burn less fat after consuming their meals than men. This results in fat storage reserves being built up around the body. It is believed that this excess fat storage and the resulting changes in a woman's body are designed to prepare us for our child-bearing years. Unfortunately, this doesn't miraculously go away once those years have passed (University of New South Wales, 2009).

THE INTERMITTENT FASTING JOURNEY OF MEN AND WOMEN

No one is going to argue that there are remarkable differences between men and women. One thing that is true for both is that fasting correctly will be beneficial in terms of optimal weight and health. As any of us who have tried to diet alongside a male counterpart can attest, that is often where the similarities end. The effects of weight-loss strategies between genders, in general, are markedly different, and men burn and discard excess fat much more quickly and efficiently than women. The physiological differences between men and women and their body's response to fasting are believed to date back to prehistoric times. During these early years, long before we had commercialized and overly processed foods to thwart attempts at weight loss, our ancestors adopted the simple yet efficient hunter-gatherer lifestyle. Before the "rules" changed and we began seeking equality and blending traditional gender roles, men hunted for food, and women gathered corn, berries, or ground nuts. It is believed that the differences in physical body size, metabolic health, and fat storage can be accredited to the hunter-gatherer lives they led.

It's All About Gender Inequality—Even in Research

In my research, I came across not only inequality in the ways that men's and women's bodies respond to intermittent fasting but in the research studies themselves. One source mentioned that the Harvard database houses at least 71 intermittent fasting studies. Of those 71 studies, only 13 mention women as test subjects. There have been zero controlled studies focusing solely on women and the effects of IF. This makes it difficult to know whether the results of the available studies and their conclusions apply to women as well as men. More gender-specific research on IF needs to be done before we can answer these questions conclusively.

Studies have shown that both men and women have a similar positive response to their IF lifestyles when adjusted to meet their individual needs. The speed at which they reach their goals may differ, but they will both get there eventually.

Studies have also shown that women generally feel the effects and benefits of intermittent fasting more quickly than men because of the shift in our metabolic state. We can feel the metabolic shift when our bodies begin burning fat instead of glucose for energy. Since men typically burn more fat than women, it takes longer for them to feel these changes.

A study using ten women and eight men was conducted in 2005 to see if there were any correlations between fasting and feelings between the genders. The study concluded that women reacted to fasting by being hungrier than men. Another study showed that men are more likely to be able to stick to a strict fasting regimen than women (Uher et al., 2006). This shouldn't discourage us from fasting; it just means putting in a little more effort to reach our desired results.

Intermittent fasting has the potential to increase triglycerides in the body as it breaks down fat, and they have been detected in the lean tissues of various test subjects. The studies have indicated that men are more likely to see a build-up of triglycerides in their liver, whereas women store them in their lean muscle (Browning et al., 2011). More research is needed to determine whether there could be any adverse health effects from this process.

Research has been done regarding the effects of IF on insulin levels and insulin resistance and the differences in impact on men and women, but the results are inconclusive. In this area, like others, more research is needed.

One thing we do know is that men and women have different hormones which affect all aspects of our bodies functioning and health. For women, our hormones affect our mood, metabolism, menstrual cycle, ovulation, hunger levels, fat storage, and more. These definitely play into our experiences with intermittent fasting and will necessitate us taking a different path than our male counterparts, whose hormones are unique to their gender and bodies' functioning. Hormones vary not only between genders but also between individuals. No woman is exactly like another, so the things that affect me and my hormones may not affect you. Again, one size doesn't fit all, and you will need to experiment to find what's best for you.

THE BOTTOM LINE

Countless women have successfully incorporated intermittent fasting into their lifestyle with no ill effects. You're unique, and your response to intermittent fasting will be as distinct as you are. Listen to your body. If you feel fantastic on an intermittent fasting protocol, terrific. If you don't, modify your protocol, take a break, or eliminate fasting altogether. IF has many positive effects on the body in addition to potential weight loss. Pay attention to how you feel in order to determine if IF is making you healthier.

Due to hormonal factors and the fact that women hold onto excess fat more readily than men, it can take time for IF to make a difference in a woman's weight. Don't get discouraged, and give this time to work. Don't obsess with a number on the scale—pay attention to body changes and physical well-being. If you have weight to lose but have not lost any weight on your IF plan after giving it time to make a difference (at least 1–2 months), try adjusting things such as the timing of your eating window, foods you are eating during your feasting window, or try tracking calories to make sure you are not taking in more than you need. Most of us will still need a calorie deficit for significant weight loss—though some women have experienced loss after adding IF without changing eating habits in other ways.

Researchers are still putting the pieces together on exactly how different types of intermittent fasting affect us and what may be the best approach for men vs. women. In the meantime, intermittent fasting, done properly, could still be an excellent fit for your lifestyle and health goals.

6

WHAT TO EXPECT IN YOUR 50S AND BEYOND AND HOW INTERMITTENT FASTING CAN HELP

The benefit of intermittent fasting over the age of 50 is a well-known phenomenon among those who make their living being fit, fierce, and fabulous at any age. The iconic Halle Berry, aged 56, has been following a time-restricted version of IF, which she combines with a ketogenic eating plan (aka the Keto diet). Halle has mentioned that she consumes only two meals a day in order to manage her diabetes. She is also active and incorporates sports and fitness such as yoga, stretching, boxing, and full-body core strength exercises.

Two other celebrities who are not shy about sharing their IF success stories and helpful hints are Jennifer Aniston and Jennifer Lopez—both aged 53. They have spoken about their journeys on television and in interviews, as well as on podcasts and other social media platforms. Lopez follows the

16:8 method. She skips breakfast, typically consumes her first meal at 1 p.m., and resumes her fast at 9 p.m. She also incorporates a cardio workout in the mornings while still fasting. In a 2019 article with Us Magazine, Jennifer Aniston said she also follows the 16:8 approach. She states that she doesn't eat any solid food in the morning. She does, however, start her day with celery juice and coffee. This would be considered "dirty fasting." There is no definitive information on what times her eating and fasting windows begin or end. All three of these women practice IF differently, yet we can all agree that they are doing something right.

PREPARING FOR YOUR 50S

I fully believe that women get better as we age. We have an appreciation for life, innumerable skills, depth of experience, and a well-rounded character that increases with every year. Women are interesting, and we are strong! It is true that some very specific challenges accompany aging; however, women over 50 can (and most likely will) find the IF lifestyle very helpful when faced with age-specific health concerns. Making IF a way of life can help us regain energy, vitality, and overall well-being.

In this next section, we will look at potential health issues we may face as we venture into our 50s and beyond. Please remember that not all of us will experience all of these—and different people will experience different levels of severity if we do develop them. This is just an overview and is meant to help you see the variety of ways IF can help, moving forward.

Menopause

I can tell you that no woman likes to hear about menopause and the side effects that accompany it. The definition of menopause is a shift in a woman's reproductive hormones, bringing an end to menstruation. This shift can wreak havoc on our bodies. That being said, it is possible to decrease the adverse effects and skip the nightmare we've heard about from the other women who have gone before us. Common side effects of hormonal changes associated with menopause include depression, mood swings, hot flashes, decreased confidence, and low self-esteem.

Studies have shown that IF is associated with decreased stress and anxiety. It also helps manage depression and can reduce the sense of hopelessness that often accompanies declining health and well-being. An increase in BDNF (a protein that promotes healthy brain function) due to IF can also improve sleep, which plays a role in mood stabilization. In addition to the chemical changes, physical body changes can increase women's self-esteem and boost confidence.

Weight Gain

This is a concern for many of us from the time we notice we have a body. For billions of women (literally, as it is believed that around 2 billion adults worldwide are overweight and more than 1 million are obese), weight is a constant struggle. The increasing pressure to conform from social media and advertising hasn't helped this. The sad reality is that the older you get, the slower your metabolism becomes—and this is often most noticeable after turning 50. To maintain your current weight, you will need to adjust your calorie intake. If your metabolism slows down and you are still consuming the same number of calories, you will find yourself gaining weight. Even an increase in exercise will often not counteract this. In general, you can't out-exercise a bad diet or one that is no longer based on your body's requirements (Elflein, 2022).

Debra Atkinson, the founder and CEO of Flipping 50, stated that a woman's body is not shy about storing fat as we age. It takes longer and a lot more effort to burn fat when we find ourselves constantly worried, stressed, or dehydrated (all of which are common as we age). She goes on to say that not only are we not burning fat as efficiently as we once did—we also tend to gain more weight around our bellies and lose our hourglass figures.

This book delves into various ways that IF helps with weight control, so we will not repeat all of them here. Suffice it to say that the very nature of IF is designed to address excess body fat and weight and does so through many methods. These include calorie reduction, fat burning through ketogenesis and autophagy, and also decreasing insulin resistance. When we are insulin resistant, our bodies store the increased sugar in our blood as fat, which makes weight loss more difficult (Wellness & Prevention, 2022).

Another thing we may notice is that the fat we are accumulating will start to find new places to settle. Where we once had evenly distributed fat on our thighs and hips, it may now find its way to our chest or belly. This redistribution generally starts happening after menopause.

Skin Changes

Age and menopause play a big part in skin health. The older we become, the less estrogen our body produces. When this happens, the body slows down collagen production, which is what keeps our skin elastic and "bouncing back." The decrease in collagen will leave the skin crepey and highlight those skin dimples lovingly referred to as cellulite.

In addition to decreased elasticity, skin starts thinning as we age. This can be caused by a variety of factors, some age-related and some due to lifestyle and environment. Sun damage, pollution, dehydration, dry climates, genetics, and side effects from certain medications all play a role in thinning skin. A skincare routine including cleansing, moisturizing, and sunscreen application helps protect skin and goes a long way toward younger-looking skin later in life. It is never too late to start, to prevent further damage.

Does an anti-inflammatory intermittent fasting lifestyle help improve dull, lifeless skin? Absolutely! Drinking lots of unsweetened water and tea can help replenish valuable fluid in the skin, reducing the look of wrinkles, improving elasticity, and even decreasing scarring. Vegetables and fruits high in water content, such as cucumber, celery, zucchini, asparagus, oranges, berries, and melon will also boost hydration and leave you with a healthy, youthful glow. Eating foods high in antioxidants (found only in plant foods) can counteract the free radicals responsible for causing wrinkles. Foods high in antioxidants will also combat sun and environmental damage, which make us look older and put us at risk for skin cancer.

Poor Eyesight

The older we get, the more difficult it is to see clearly. This can be attributed to both external and physical factors, as well as chronic metabolic diseases and their effects on vision. The ability to see in low light decreases, as does depth perception. Most of us who drive at night can attest to this. Another age, hormonal, and medication-related change is dry eyes—tear production decreases, which can cause discomfort and difficulty focusing vision.

Believe it or not, intermittent fasting can help improve your vision and decrease further vision changes or degeneration. It can also reverse the effects of many metabolic health issues that contribute to poor eyesight. Intermittent fasting can lower blood pressure as well as blood sugar, both of which improve blood flow to the eyes. Diabetes is a considerable risk factor for vision impairment or blindness, and mitigating or eliminating symptoms of diabetes can also eliminate the risk of your vision deteriorating. In addition, the ketone bodies generated by fasting can decrease eye inflammation and oxidative stress. Adding an anti-inflammatory diet to the mix will also add antioxidants and vital nutrients that protect and heal eye damage, like lutein, vitamin C, vitamin E, and zinc. These are plentiful in green leafy vegetables, fruits, nuts, seeds, and other plant foods (Feng et al., 2022).

Dry Mouth

Women over 50 will often struggle with dry mouth. This can be attributed to chronic health problems and autoimmune disorders such as Sjogren's syndrome or diabetes, as well as their medication effects. Dry mouth can also be caused by inadequate nutrition or dehydration.

Intermittent fasting can help with dry mouth by improving metabolic health and decreasing the symptoms of chronic health disorders and the amount of medication needed to control them. Many people have found that they can reduce or eliminate medications as their health improves (but only in consultation with a medical care provider). The increased fluid intake associated with IF and water-packed anti-inflammatory foods can also alleviate this condition. Antioxidant-rich ginger stimulates saliva production and is a great addition to the diet for those with dry mouth.

Low Bone Density

The National Osteoporosis Foundation has identified that young women will experience an increase in their bone density until they reach 30. After age 30, bone density will gradually decrease. Once women reach menopause, they lose approximately 0.5% to 1.5% of their bone density yearly. Individuals who have not included aerobic weight-bearing exercise in their routines, have not consumed a vitamin D-rich diet, or have not taken calcium supplements may find that they are losing an average of 3% to 5% bone density a year. This will make bones weak, brittle, and prone to fracture (Downing, 2022).

While there is not enough research to conclude that IF can reverse osteoporosis, animal studies have shown that fasting may improve the bone remodeling process by stimulating the secretion of parathyroid hormone (PTH). Other ways to slow or possibly reverse osteoporosis include getting regular exercise, eliminating alcohol and highly processed, sugary foods from the diet, and eating foods rich in calcium and Vitamin D. When paired with IF, you will be well on your way to strong, healthy bones (Alrowaili et al., 2021).

Musculoskeletal Issues

Debra Atkinson, whom I referred to earlier, has noted that a woman's muscle mass shows a remarkable peak in their mid-twenties. She also cautions that a decrease in muscle mass will occur as we age. Along with an expected slowing of endocrine function, decreased physical activity and poor nutrition add to this process.

Joint and muscle pains are something many of us face as we age. We begin to experience changes in joint lubrication and cushioning, which can delay recovery. This is especially true when we have repeated stress on our joints. This will result in muscle pain and stiffness and can lead to chronic arthritis.

While arthritis is common in older populations, it is not limited to seniors. Athletes or highly active individuals put a lot of strain and impact on their joints, and the same can be said for those who carry around a few (or more) extra pounds. Arthritis is the build-up of inflammation from prolonged damage to your joints and cartilage. While it is a painful and sometimes debilitating condition, it is often manageable with the help of diet and exercise.

Intermittent fasting can help with musculoskeletal issues in various ways. First, weight loss will result in less pressure and wear-and-tear being put on the joints. It can also reduce inflammation, alleviating the pain associated with these conditions and preventing worsening. IF contributes to an increase in lean muscle mass and, when combined with weight-bearing exercises, can reduce the risk of muscle loss.

Declining Libido

Here we are, back at the hormones. As we age, our hormone levels decrease. When testosterone and growth hormones become depleted, it affects our libido, and our sex drive plummets. A decrease in estrogen also affects the lubrication of the vagina, which can further suppress our libido out of fear of pain during intercourse. Poor self-esteem due to increased weight, or other body changes related to aging, can have a further negative effect. These things combined can negatively impact our relationships and our mental health. But there is hope.

For many people, men and women alike, intermittent fasting increases libido. This could be the result of changing hormone levels but is likely due to multiple factors. One hypothesis is that during fasting, when the body's blood is not needed for digestion, it travels to other areas of the body, including the genitals, and increased circulation stimulates the sex drive. When paired with healthy eating, the improvement in nutrition and hydration can also play a part in both improved circulation and increased lubrication. One of the most significant contributors to an improved libido is likely the boost in self-confidence and self-esteem that comes with adopting a new lifestyle and the body changes happening as a result. Face it; when we feel better, we feel sexier. And when we feel sexy, we are sexy!

Lactose Intolerance

Lactose intolerance is something that, even if tolerated earlier in life, can develop as we age. We can either develop a new case of lactose intolerance, or an existing case can worsen over time. Symptoms can include gas, bloating, diarrhea, stomach cramps, nausea, and vomiting. If you cannot tolerate dairy products (and most of them are not recommended in an anti-inflammatory diet anyway), you can get your calcium from soy milk, leafy greens, tofu, edamame, and other calcium-rich plant foods.

I can find no human studies addressing intermittent fasting and its effect on lactose intolerance, but one source cites an animal study showing that IF increases human growth hormone (HGH), which boosts lactase production in the body. Lactase is an enzyme that breaks down lactose in our bodies. In a personal blog, the author also states that her lactose intolerance was cured once she began IF. If following an anti-inflammatory diet along with fasting, lactose won't be an issue, as dairy in most forms is considered inflammatory, and plant-based substitutes are encouraged (Prescott, 2020).

Cognitive Decline

The sad reality is that the less we use our brains as we get older, the more our brains can weaken. This can happen as we retire and leave our challenging jobs for an easier, more relaxed way of life. This underuse causes symptoms that manifest as memory loss, decreased cognition, slowed reaction times, changes in judgment, and poor body awareness.

Intermittent fasting is beneficial on many cognitive fronts. It has been linked to better outcomes for stroke survivors, prevention of Alzheimer's disease, slowing of the aging process, and more. It is believed that changes to the metabolic processes during fasting can boost neuroplasticity in the brain, which protects against disease and injury and maximizes brain function. Exercise and a healthy diet also play a part in enhancing memory and cognition. Intermittent fasting, combined with healthy lifestyle changes, gives us the best chance of maintaining our brain health for as long as possible.

Dental Concerns

Dental issues don't always come to mind when we think of problems associated with aging, but people over age 50 are at increased risk for periodontal disease, eroded tooth enamel, and cavities. Lifelong poor eating habits can contribute to these conditions, as can medication use.

Intermittent fasting has been shown to decrease inflammation and, as a result, can also decrease the instance of gum and periodontal disease. Reduction in the intake of highly processed, sugary foods due to adopting an IF lifestyle can also reduce the risk of further tooth damage and cavity production. As mentioned before, improving health markers could also lead to fewer medications, which can improve inflammation, bleeding, and mouth ulcers.

Suppressed Immune System

Aging affects everything, and the immune system is no exception. As we age, our bodies produce less of the cells designed to fight disease and infection, thus leaving us at a higher risk of getting sick. Healing can be slower, and our bodies no longer recognize threats to the system as effectively as they did when we were young. That makes us vulnerable to developing not only infections but also diseases such as cancer.

Intermittent fasting can boost and assist the immune system in many ways. First, it decreases inflammation, which helps the body's immune system work more efficiently. It can fight actual threats rather than working against itself. Autophagy, as I have mentioned several times already, is responsible for cleaning and removing damaged cells. Valter Longo, a scientist, and researcher at USC, found in a 2014 study that fasting can ultimately increase white blood cell counts, which help fight infection and other diseases. He states that fasting can do a kind of reset for the immune system (Salzberg, 2020).

Digestive Concerns

The older we become, the more difficult it is to keep our digestive systems happy. We may experience issues such as constipation, excessive gas, or bloating. Our bodies are changing, and the foods we once loved may not love us in return. As we age, the stomach begins to limit its production of acid, which assists with digestion and absorption of medication and supplements. This may affect bowel movements and cause heartburn or acid reflux.

Intermittent fasting can benefit digestion in several ways. First, the rest provided to our systems during fasting, even for just a few hours, can greatly benefit overall digestion and decrease gas, bloating, and other issues. It is also believed that IF can improve gut microbiome and reduce gut permeability. Intermittent fasting also shows promise in healing more severe disorders of the GI system, such as irritable bowel syndrome (IBS).

Breast Cancer

This is a disease that doesn't discriminate based on age but affects one in eight women, according to research by the National Cancer Institute. The research has established that a woman in her 30s has a 0.5% chance of being diagnosed with breast cancer over the next ten years. Even more concerning, a woman in her 60s has a 3.5% chance of being diagnosed later on in life—that puts the statistics at one in twenty-eight women (National Cancer Institute, 2018). Metabolic disturbances put women at an even greater risk of developing breast cancer.

Intermittent fasting can help mitigate metabolic disturbances, and by reducing insulin levels and body fat, IF may also reduce the risk of breast cancer. Low-calorie diets have also been shown to prevent cancer and improve breast cancer treatment outcomes.

Our Aging Cells

Our bodies are made up of cells, tissues, muscles, skin, and organs. It is only natural that our old cells are recycled or made redundant to make space for new ones. As we age, our bodies have a harder time doing this. The damage to our cells can be exacerbated by exposure to harsh medications and treatments such as radiation therapy, chemotherapy, or exposure to sunlight.

Autophagy to the rescue! One of the best components of our body's healing process is autophagy, and IF boosts this process. It allows our bodies to take old, damaged cells and break them down so that they can be either removed, or recycled and remodeled to work more efficiently.

Other 50s Setbacks

We have examined a long list of general body changes accompanying aging and how intermittent fasting can help with each. Now let's look at a few more specific issues that we may or may not encounter. Though I won't go into how intermittent fasting can help with each one, rest assured that it can in most cases! If you are struggling with any of these, I suggest you do some research on your own about how IF may or may not affect them.

- **High cholesterol**: Estrogen assists with keeping the walls of the arteries supple and offers aid in keeping both good and bad cholesterol in check—menopause will deplete you of your already decreased estrogen levels, and high cholesterol may result.
- **Risk of heart disease**: It is believed that menopausal women are at a higher risk of suffering heart attacks because of the reduction of estrogen; following an

anti-inflammatory diet that is rich in whole grains, fruit, and vegetables will help protect your heart.

- **High blood pressure**: As has been previously mentioned, the decrease in estrogen will affect women's blood vessels—our hearts are inclined to work harder to compensate for our age, and in the long run, this may lead to high blood pressure.
- **Insomnia**: Sleep disorders such as restless leg syndrome or sleep apnea may lead to difficulty sleeping. Other conditions, both physical and mental such as anxiety or depression, can also play a role. Age-related lifestyle changes such as napping or decreased physical exercise can change sleep patterns and lead to insomnia.
- **Body odor**: Changing hormones as a result of menopause (mainly a decrease in estrogen and a resulting increase in testosterone) can lead to bacteria in our sweat and will affect the way we smell. This can also lead to acne in later years.
- **Loss of taste**: People tend to experience a decrease in smell and taste as they age. To a degree, this is normal but may also be the result of medications or physiological disorders such as allergies or sinus problems. Decreased sense of smell and taste can be problematic in terms of weight, as it is possible to overeat while trying to get satisfaction from our food.

THE BENEFITS OF INTERMITTENT FASTING IN YOUR 50S AND BEYOND

This chapter section summarizes what IF can do to help combat, address, or resolve age-related or general health issues. Everything has previously been mentioned, but it is always good to have a concise list to refer back to. Intermittent fasting:

Manages Nutritional Requirements

- assists with weight loss
- helps to reduce or get rid of belly fat
- restricts calories, which is beneficial for both weight loss and reducing the risk of cancer growth
- lowers insulin resistance
- regulates the circadian rhythm, which promotes better glucose tolerance and better sleep
- boosts brain function by increasing BDNF expression (which is a protein that serves as a sort of "fertilizer" or "miracle-grow" for the brain and promotes alertness and energy). It also helps promote restful sleep
- increases cell turnover—autophagy helps "clean out" damaged cells and increases healing

Reduces the Risks of Physical Illnesses

- reduces diabetes
- reduces digestive issues by allowing your digestive system to rest during fasting periods
- reduces inflammation, which is a condition that can lead to various diseases
- reduces blood pressure
- lowers bad LDL cholesterol levels
- helps prevent osteoporosis
- helps prevent and manage arthritis
- is associated with better outcomes for stroke survivors
- helps protect against cancer
- helps protect against multiple sclerosis
- may help to prevent Alzheimer's disease
- helps prevent and correct vision problems
- may slow kidney disease

Improves Well-Being and Mental Health Issues Related to Menopause and Hormonal Changes

- decreases stress and anxiety
- helps to manage depression
- helps improve self-esteem
- helps boost confidence
- decreases the sense of hopelessness associated with declining physical well-being

Improves Lifestyle

- promotes better sleep
- improves energy levels
- increases libido and improves sex life
- cultivates a greater appreciation for food

Additional Benefits

- improves skin quality and texture
- helps with dental health

MY STORY OF FASTING AND HEALING

I woke up one day, during my 49th year, to the certainty that I was dying. My sister had died at the age of 52 from an auto-immune disorder, and I became convinced that the same was happening to me. At that time, I had lived in a remote village in Nepal for four years. Life in the village is physically demanding, and I was increasingly unable to tolerate it. I washed my clothes, dishes, and body in a river. It was back-breaking work. The "toilets" were nothing more than squat holes in the ground, and in order to use them, you had to squat all the way down and then be able to get back up afterward (the hardest part)! All interactions with others took place sitting cross-legged on the ground or dirt floor. I had to haul 70-pound jugs of water up to the house from the stream for cooking and everyday use. To get anywhere from my house, I had to walk straight up or down a mountain gorge on treacherous paths to a small dirt road above or below.

There was nothing physically easy in my days or in my life. Increasingly, my legs were getting heavier and less mobile. They often felt like they had lead in them. Walking on easy terrain, much less mountain paths, was becoming harder and harder. I had constant pain in my legs from hip to toe with no apparent source and no relief. This was affecting not only my waking hours but also my sleep. I just couldn't get comfortable. I realized that if something didn't change quickly, I would no longer be able to live the life and do the work that I so desperately loved and wanted to continue. I began a journey of self-discovery and inquiry into what was causing my pain. I prayed that I could prove wrong my theory that I was dying.

Around the time that this journey began, I turned 50. Completely unhappy with who I had become and the limitations my body was experiencing, I decided to take control of the things I could control, and the first hurdle was losing weight. I knew that no matter what was wrong with me, I would benefit from losing pounds and taking unnecessary pressure off my legs and joints. I read about the positive effects of both an anti-inflammatory diet and intermittent fasting, and I went all-in. I switched to only eating foods on the "acceptable" list of the anti-inflammatory diet I found online, cutting out meat, dairy, and other commonly inflammatory foods. I started eating only between the hours of 10 a.m. and 6 p.m. Something amazing happened. Before this, I had hit a weight plateau. There had actually been many plateaus, and they had become higher and higher with each passing year.

No matter what I did, I could not get under those plateaus. The current plateau had been long-standing, and I had not been under it in what seemed like forever. And then, I switched to a plant-based diet and IF. For literally the first time in 15 years, I dropped below that plateau. In just 11 days, I had lost 15 pounds. I knew that all 15 pounds couldn't be fat, but that proved to me that my body was holding on to a massive amount of inflammation and that this wasn't beneficial or healthy for me. My swollen legs shrank down two sizes in two weeks. The changes in my body in such a short time motivated me to add in even more healthy activities in an attempt to maximize the results.

After renewed hope that I could, in fact, make positive changes in my body, I decided to add exercise. I joined an online program that promised to "shred away pounds and shred your body" into some form of a goddess. With this group came an online forum where women post before and after photos of themselves in their underwear as they progress. It was meant to be encouraging, assuring each other that we could see a difference and it wasn't a lost cause. I posted my own before photos and received a comment from another woman in the group. She said, "I am a physical therapist specializing in treating women with Lipedema, and I wonder if you have been evaluated for it because you look to me like you have it." My first response, as always, was, "No, I'm just fat." That is the narrative I had heard and had been telling myself for years. I am a medical person, however, and in my skepticism, I looked into it. I was stunned. Within 15 minutes of looking at other women's photos and reading the information I could find online, I knew what was wrong with me. Suddenly my whole life made sense.

Lipedema is not yet well understood and is primarily unrecognized, even by medical professionals. It is an inflammatory disorder with lymphatic and connective tissue components, resulting in large, swollen, hardened, and painful fat deposits on the hips and legs (primarily) and sometimes the arms and other areas of the body. The condition also causes a lot of fibrosis, or scarring, within the affected tissues, exacerbating the pain. The fat itself is not "normal" fat and is entirely unaffected by diet or exercise—meaning that once it is there, it is impossible to reduce without surgery to remove the diseased fat tissue. I was both relieved to have an answer and despairing that there was "nothing I could do" to improve my situation. Through even more research and listening to the stories of other brave women who had walked this road before me, I determined that there were ways to minimize the effects of Lipedema and maximize my health condition even if I couldn't cure the disease. Healing doesn't have to be total to be worthwhile. So I set out to heal myself, determined to be as healthy and strong as possible. I would learn that the best way to do that was to heal myself through food.

As I delved deeper and deeper into what an anti-inflammatory diet looked like, I made the decision to further eliminate other middle-of-the-road inflammatory foods. Those on the "sometimes acceptable" or "eat in moderation" lists. That eliminated all meat, dairy, gluten, sugar, alcohol, and processed foods. I switched to a strict whole-foods-plant-based way of eating. I still had a myriad of fantastic foods to choose from; fruits, vegetables, beans, legumes, nuts, seeds, greens, grains, etc... I made the decision to only put high-level anti-oxidant-rich foods into my body, and the results were astounding. Remember that weight plateau? I blazed past it. Though I wasn't able to lose the "lipedema fat," I lost both regular fat and fluid retention due to inflammation. Both my size and my pain began to decrease. I lost 38 pounds in under a year. For the first time in literally as long as I could remember, I was a "normal" size for my height. The pain in my legs went from a constant 6 or higher on a 0-10 scale to a manageable 2 or 3 most days. The heaviness lessened, and my mobility increased. I was healing and could feel it in every part of my body and life.

While the plant-based diet made an amazing difference in how I felt and my weight loss, let's not forget the intermittent fasting. I thought, at first, that I had found the key to health in the diet, and slowly but surely, I eased off of the intermittent fasting. First, I added breakfast back into the lineup, shortening my fasting window to a mere 12–14 hours. Then I found myself allowing myself a snack at bedtime on those days I found myself hungry at night. Eventually, though plant-based eating remained, the IF did not. It made a difference in how I felt. I gained some of the weight back. I had more episodes of unexplained heaviness in my legs and leg swelling at the end of the day. I was overall more bloated, and not just in my legs. It also affected my mood and my energy level. I am sure there were multiple factors at play, such as increased calories due to the elimination of fasting times and more hours in which to eat them, but it was more than that. The weight gain was not enough to account for the increase in pain and the overall decrease in my sense of well-being.

I was experiencing low-level inflammation that could only be explained by the elimination of fasting. Both the eating and the fasting were working together in a way that was larger than the sum of their individual parts. It was almost magical. I added IF back into my self-care routine, and all of the original benefits returned. It is important to note that I have also, at times, tried IF with a more standard diet (adding in gluten, alcohol, sugar, or some animal products), particularly when traveling or socializing, and the results were the same. The IF on its own was not as effective as the combination of the two, and when I switched back to a plant-strong way of eating, my symptoms significantly improved or resolved altogether.

So there you have it—plant-based eating and intermittent fasting are beneficial and can potentially heal a myriad of what ails you. You can do them individually or in combination, and you will receive benefits and healing regardless. That said, as with most things, the more diligent you are in sticking to these principles, and the more you can combine them in a way that works for your life, the better. You will get out of it more than you put into it because it is more about adding healthy habits than eliminating harmful ones. You have control. With these tools, you can start rediscovering that healthier, more vital YOU. Like me, you can be a healthier version of yourself than you were prior to turning 50. Isn't that exciting? Why wait?!

FIFTY AND FABULOUS... HELP ME SPREAD THE WORD!

"Aging is not lost youth but a new stage of opportunity and strength." — Betty Friedan

Did you know that taking a positive view of aging is enough on its own to boost your health? And that's before you take control of your physical health and fitness!

A study conducted by researchers at Harvard T.H. Chan School of Public Health found that people with the most positive view of aging were at a lower risk of developing conditions like heart disease, diabetes, and cancer. They also had better brain health and were more likely to have healthier habits.

It's natural for many people to panic as they approach the 50-year milestone, but taking a positive approach and putting your health front and center is key to launching into the next phase of your life with energy and vitality.

I want to help as many people as I can to realize that and take the necessary steps to make their transition into later life as positive as possible... Thereby staying younger and healthier for longer.

This is your opportunity to help me do that.

By leaving a review of this book on Amazon, you'll show other women approaching their 50s where they can find the guidance they need to take charge of their health through fasting and adopting a positive attitude to aging.

Simply by letting other readers know how this book has helped you and what they can expect to find inside it, you'll help make this bumpy transition period a little easier for someone else – and help them see that intermittent fasting isn't as difficult as it sounds.

Thank you so much for helping me reach more people. It's a privilege to grow older... and when we can embrace it with optimum health, it has so much to offer us.

Scan the QR code below for a quick review!

7

FEAST MODE—HOW TO MAKE THE MOST OF YOUR EATING WINDOW

The last chapter was intense, with lots of heavy information. I want to lighten things up with this chapter and start with some fun and interesting facts about food.

I came across an article written by Joanna Fantozzi for the Insider online publication titled *Amazing Things You Didn't Know About Food*. Think of this as a culinary *Ripley's Believe It or Not*.

- Potatoes were used to test the activity of radio and wireless signals on airplanes; because of their water content and chemical makeup, they reflect and absorb these signals in the same way that humans do and can be used as stand-ins!

- Bananas are technically classified as berries, while strawberries are just fruit—botanists have weighed in and said that fruit should come from a single flower (and have seeds), and what we know as berries come from single flowers that consist of a singular ovary and have multiple seeds. Strawberries, raspberries, and blackberries actually come from a flower with multiple ovaries, so don't count.
- Chocolates were (are) a hot commodity, but the Aztecs took their love of chocolate to the next level when they demanded that individuals pay their taxes with used cocoa beans!
- Individuals once believed tomatoes were toxic because 18th-century Europeans discovered that aristocrats often died after consuming the "poison apples." They didn't know that it was actually due to the pewter tableware they were using, which leached lead into their food from the acidity of the tomatoes.
- Peanut butter is rich in carbon, and scientists at the Bayerisches Geoinstitut discovered that it is possible to turn plain, simple peanut butter into—diamonds! The formula includes extracting oxygen from the carbon dioxide in the peanut butter and inflicting intense pressure on the remaining carbon (Fantozzi, 2020).

THE "RULES" FOR INTERMITTENT FASTING

In my opinion, one of the first rules of IF should be to become reacquainted with food. This is a journey where you will learn to appreciate your food and not view it as the enemy. Society has been telling us for so long that we "shouldn't eat this because it causes that" or that consuming too much of that will be a "moment on the lips, and a lifetime on the hips." This has done nothing but increase our anxiety surrounding eating. Intermittent fasting will teach you to appreciate your food again and help you heal your body and mind. Remember that IF is not a diet; it is a change in how you approach your meals' timing. Let's go through some of the "rules" that apply to IF and how you can transform your lifestyle into something comfortable and amazing by following them.

Intermittent fasting doesn't limit what you can eat, and the focus is primarily on when you eat. That being said, IF is not an invitation to eat anything and everything during all of your eating windows. Foods such as ice cream, candy, pastries, chips, cookies, or chocolates should be enjoyed sparingly (if at all) and saved for special occasions. You will want to avoid unhealthy foods and opt for lower-calorie foods that will offer you sustenance and keep you feeling fuller for longer—that is when you will reap the maximum results from your IF journey. Remember, nothing tastes better than healthy feels!

One of the best pieces of advice I can share is that you should plan balanced meals that will offer maximum benefits for your overall health and well-being. We know that IF is about eating during a specific time frame, so you want to optimize your health by ensuring that you make healthy food choices and meet your nutritional requirements daily. Focus on consuming foods rich in protein, fiber, complex carbs, and healthy fats from plant-based sources.

Clean Eating

I introduced you to the Warrior Diet in Chapter 4, where I touched on clean versus dirty eating. In my opinion, eating clean is the key! Clean eating is a term that the dietary community has adopted, aimed at educating individuals to choose less processed foods, focus on whole foods that have not been preserved with chemicals, and opt for natural or organically grown food. This may not always be possible, but there is a benefit to striving to reach this goal. In this day and age, convenience (and societal pressure) thwart our health plans, which is the cycle we are trying to break.

Helpful Hints and Tips for Clean Eating

I would like to offer some helpful tips on how you can eat clean and achieve optimal health benefits by making a few changes here and a few tweaks there.

- Increase your consumption of fresh fruit and vegetables.

- Limit processed foods such as deli meat, hotdogs, or "heat and eat" pre-cooked meals.
- Limit your consumption of refined carbs, which include bread, cookies, pastries, or pasta, and replace them with whole-grain options.
- Limit or eliminate your consumption of alcohol.
- Minimize or eliminate your consumption of sugar-laden beverages or food.
- Limit or minimize the use of oil, which contains 120 calories per tablespoon—oil is responsible for trauma to arteries and inflammation; sparingly use plant-based oils such as avocado or olive oil, if any.
- Use vegetable proteins instead of animal or processed proteins when cooking.
- Steer clear of snack bags of chips, cookies, or crackers. Try to eat foods that come from the ground and not from a package.
- Water, water, water—the primary beverage of choice.
- Know what you are putting in your mouth. Read the labels. Chemicals, sugar, salt, oil, and a vast array of things that aren't actually food are hiding everywhere.

ANTI-INFLAMMATORY DIET

While our bodies need inflammation to fight illnesses and to protect us from viral or bacterial infections, some individuals produce an excess of inflammation which can cause severe health concerns. The anti-inflammatory diet protects your body against these high levels of inflammation and decreases the likelihood of developing diseases such as rheumatoid arthritis, cellulitis, or pneumonia (Pahwa & Jialal, 2019).

What does an anti-inflammatory diet entail? This diet's essential components are foods rich in nutrients and antioxidants. Begin by consuming whole foods, which will begin the process of reducing inflammation throughout your body. The anti-inflammatory diet is rich in vegetables, fatty fish, whole fruit, legumes, and whole grains—it is preferable to steer clear of processed foods. This diet will give your body everything it needs to prevent inflammatory attacks, such as vitamins, minerals, fiber, omega-3 fatty acids, and antioxidants.

The Benefits of the Anti-Inflammatory Diet

The information in this section is courtesy of an interview with a registered dietician and nutritionist, Nancy Park, who works with the Henry Ford Health Organization. Nancy states that someone struggling with chronic inflammation may compare the pain to a fire burning inside their body. Anyone who has ever had acid reflux may sympathize. Now imagine that pain being everywhere inside you. Below are some benefits of an anti-inflammatory diet and how they can potentially transform your life.

- The natural properties in the food previously mentioned will help to soothe the inflammation in your body, therefore acting as a preventative measure against various health conditions and diseases.
- It will lower your risk of inflammatory illnesses and diseases such as obesity, auto-immune diseases, IBS, arthritis, heart conditions, and Alzheimer's disease.
- It will improve your overall physical health.
- You will experience less pain in affected areas.
- It will increase your mobility.
- Your life expectancy will increase.
- It will slow down the aging process.
- It will prevent cancer (Henry Ford Health Staff, 2020).

Anti-Inflammatory Diet Food List

The key to following an anti-inflammatory diet is knowing which foods to eat and which to avoid. The following food list is an example of the types of food your inflamed body may find soothing and healing. The upside is that they are both nutritious and delicious. Just a reminder that you don't have to be diagnosed with an inflammatory disease to follow this diet—it is a wholesome way of eating that offers endless benefits and prevents future diseases and conditions.

- **Fresh vegetables**: No restrictions, but make sure to consume at least four or five servings daily of vegetables of varying colors and types, such as dark and leafy greens, beetroot, and cauliflower.

- **Fresh fruit**: The recommendation is three to four servings a day—no fruit juices. Smoothies are okay if they contain whole, ground fruit.
- **Fatty fish**: Omega-3 essential fats include salmon, trout, sardines, tuna, and mackerel.
- **Herbs and spices**: For example, turmeric, cinnamon, basil, ginger, thyme, and oregano.
- **Healthy fats**: Avocado, olives, tofu, nuts, seeds, and fatty fish. *The use of oil is controversial, as it can also cause inflammation. If using, stick to avocado oil, seed or nut oils, or extra virgin olive oil, and use sparingly.
- **Nuts and seeds**: Hemp and chia seeds, walnuts, pistachios, pine nuts, and almonds. A cautionary note for those wanting to lose weight—nuts and seeds are high in fat and calories and should be eaten in moderation. Pay close attention to portion sizes.
- **Whole grains**: Quinoa, buckwheat, amaranth, brown rice, and millet. Whole wheat, rye, and barley are also whole grains but contain gluten, which is inflammatory for some people.
- **Legumes and beans**: Black beans, red kidney beans, pinto beans, lentils, black-eyed peas, and chickpeas.
- **Beverages**: Organic coffee, herbal teas, green tea, and water.

Foods You Should Steer Clear Of

We live in a world of convenience. It is often easier, quicker, and sometimes cheaper to buy processed food. Or maybe you want to multitask and run through the drive-through while running errands. Life is busier and crazier than ever, and we are often just looking for the easy answer. Unfortunately, these grab-and-go foods we are reaching for are usually high in saturated fat, sodium, and sugar and are considerable contributors to both obesity and cardiovascular disease. Have you ever taken a moment to see how you feel after eating something highly processed? Your body must work overtime to digest that food, and it has to use the anti-inflammatory systems in place to counteract that meal's side effects. Instead of healing your body, the food you ate is hurting it, and your body is working overtime to undo the damage you have done. The reality of the situation is that our bodies are constantly playing catch-up when we eat for convenience and not health.

Let's look at a list of inflammatory foods to try and avoid. See this as a challenge, and if you aren't comfortable going all-in from the start, try to eliminate at least one item a week (or whatever you decide is right for you).

- **Processed meats**: Deli and lunch meats, bacon, and hotdogs.
- **Deep-fried foods**: Donuts and churros.

- **Whole milk and whole-fat dairy**: Milk, cream, ice cream, and full-fat cheese.
- **Refined carbs and sugar**: White bread, sugar-laden breakfast cereals, candy, soda, cookies, and high fructose corn syrup—these will all cause a spike in your blood sugar levels, which in turn awakens inflammation.
- **Alcohol**: Dry red wine is permitted in small quantities—not more than 4 ounces per day.
- **Trans fats**: Baked goods, deep-fried foods, and fast food.
- **Processed snacks**: Cookies, chips, and crackers.
- **Allergens to be avoided**: There are eight major allergens found in our food groups, which include soybeans, tree nuts, peanuts, milk, eggs, shellfish, fish, and wheat. Pay attention to how you feel after eating these foods, and eliminate if you react negatively to them.

TRANSITION TO PLANT-BASED NUTRITION

Based on a study conducted between 2014 and 2018, the popularity of plant-based eating showed a massive 600% increase among Americans. The driving forces behind changing to plant-based nutrition were for health, animal welfare, and reducing the environmental footprint (Clem & Barthel, 2021).

A plant-based diet is an anti-inflammatory way of eating that eliminates all animal sources (i.e., meat, dairy, and in some cases, honey). It is comprised of fresh fruit and vegetables, nuts, seeds, whole grains, and legumes. It also eliminates highly processed foods, so your diet will likely be healthier and lower in calories. The food list above in the anti-inflammatory diet section is the same for the plant-based diet, minus the fatty fish. Most people following a whole food plant-based diet also eliminate oil for added health benefits.

The Benefits of Plant-Based Nutrition

The benefits of a plant-based anti-inflammatory way of eating are similar to those of the regular anti-inflammatory diet, with a few additions. A plant-based lifestyle

- reduces inflammation.
- reduces the carbon footprint.
- improves kidney function.
- lowers the risk of type 2 diabetes.
- reduces the risk of heart disease.
- lowers the levels of "bad" cholesterol.
- reduces the risk of dementia and cognitive impairment.
- improves gut health.
- aids with weight loss.
- increases your lifespan.

- adds compassion to your lifestyle—no harm to animals or the environment to provide your nutrition (Alexander, 2019).

Incorporating Anti-Inflammatory or Plant-Based Diets Into the Intermittent Fasting Lifestyle

Many people have asked if they can do intermittent fasting and an anti-inflammatory diet simultaneously, and the answer is YES! That is the beauty of intermittent fasting—its versatility and flexibility. As I mentioned earlier, one of the few rules of intermittent fasting focuses on time-restricted eating and not the actual foods themselves. Because of this, IF can be used with absolutely any dietary regimen. I am also aware that many people that do intermittent fasting also adhere to a ketogenic way of eating. If that is you, I want to encourage you to keep reading and consider steering your Keto diet in a more plant-based direction. This will ensure that you get optimal nutrition and that your body gets the benefits of the multitude of healing antioxidants found only in plants. For more information on this, check out Dr. Will Cole's book *Ketotarian: The Mostly Plant-Based Plan to Burn Fat, Boost Your Energy, Crush Your Cravings, and Calm Inflammation*. I think that title speaks for itself!

With a shortened eating window each day, and subsequent decrease in the amount of food you're eating, it is essential to ensure you are consuming all of the necessary nutrients your body needs. The upside to a plant-based, anti-inflammatory diet is that everything you put in your mouth will be loaded with healthy nutrients to fuel your body and help it heal. Make sure to include a variety of foods, and have whole, natural plant-based protein, fats, and complex carbohydrates with each meal, and you should have all your bases covered.

Calories are important, especially to those of us who are in our 50s or beyond. I have heard many people who practice IF promise that you can consume whatever you want and still lose weight—and in many instances, this just isn't true. As we age, our metabolisms do decline, and the truth is that we may need to count our calories. The upside to both the time-limited eating nature of IF and the inclusion of a plant-based anti-inflammatory diet is that these two things combined generally lead to an organic decrease in calories when compared to eating the same quantities of foods from the standard American diet (SAD), and eating them all day long. Calorie counting isn't mandatory, nor even essential, but if you find that you aren't getting the results that you desire, or if you feel tired, weak, or light-headed while doing IF, it is a good idea to follow your calorie intake and expenditure for a while to see if you are, in fact, getting too many or too few calories as compared to what you are burning.

You will likely lose weight with a calorie deficit, but don't be too eager to drop pounds quickly. I realize that's easier said than done because when we find something that works, we want it to work NOW. But remember that if you cut your calories too drastically, you run the genuine risk of slowing your metabolism when you want to give it a boost. With drastic and prolonged calorie restriction, you may even permanently damage your metabolism and not be able to bring it back up to its baseline. Then, if you ever begin eating a "normal" amount of food or stop fasting, you will gain your weight back. Instead, it is healthier to aim for a 500-calorie deficit daily, below your energy needs. This will allow you to lose approximately one pound of fat a week and spare your lean muscle. It will also boost your metabolism instead of slowing it. Remember to choose foods that will satiate your appetite, such as fiber-rich, whole, and protein-packed foods (such as legumes and beans), that will ensure you stay fuller, longer.

CALORIE COUNTERS

We live in a world that relies on digital devices to think for us, which makes our lives a lot easier. That is definitely true with online calorie counters and apps. I remember the days when I had to look up each food's calorie count in a book and then do the math myself at the end of the day. Times have changed! I want to share a list of food/nutrition trackers and calorie counters that you can download to any digital device to help you prepare for your IF journey. These also track your activity or exercise and give you a running count of the calories and nutrients you are consuming and the number of calories you are burning. Many applications have monthly paid subscriptions, but most offer a basic free version as well. A word of warning—as with all things digital these days, the advertisements may be a little overwhelming.

Let's get you sorted:

- **MyFitnessPal**: $19.99 per month, $79.99 per year, or the basic version is free
- **Lose It!**: $39.99 per year, or the basic version is free
- **FatSecret**: Free
- **Cronometer**: $49.99 per year, or the basic version is free
- **Noom**: $199 per year
- **Lifesum**: $9.99 per month, $24.99 for three months, or $49.99 per year, or the basic version is free
- **MyNetDiary**: $8.99 per month, $23.99 for three months, or $59.99 per year, or the basic version is free
- **Calory**: $14.99 per year, or the basic version is free
- **Fitbit**: $8.99 per month, $23.99 for three months, or $59.99 per year, or the basic version is free. The premium version of Fitbit is $10 per month or $80 per year

8

MOVE IT OR LOSE IT! MIXING IF WITH EXERCISE AND SUPPLEMENTS

It's bad enough that we have to pay closer attention to our diets as we age, but now I'm bringing up exercise?! First, the good news. In order to do intermittent fasting, adding exercise is not mandatory. You will still reap multitudes of benefits just by fasting alone. I want to stress, however, that those benefits will be exponentially greater if you do. We have all heard phrases like, "Move it or lose it!" and "Motion is lotion." That is so, so true—especially after 50. Let's answer some common questions surrounding exercise and IF, such as, "Are they safe to combine? Which exercises are best when practicing IF?" and more.

As we have seen before with Jennifer Lopez, Halle Berry, and Jennifer Aniston, some of the most well-known celebrities practice IF and exercise together. Before we move into the specifics of incorporating exercise into your own IF lifestyle, let's take a look at another beautiful, healthy, over-50 celebrity who wholeheartedly recommends this lifestyle. She is an actress, fitness personality, and former co-host of *Dancing With the Stars*—Brooke Burke!

A quick trip to the Google image gallery when you type in Brooke's name will see her posing in a two-piece bikini with a fine-toned body and flat stomach—at 50. Various news publications have interviewed her to find out her secret. The mother of four attributes her slender figure and toned body to intermittent fasting. She was quoted in the Daily Mail as saying, "It is one of the easiest ways to lose weight" (Marks, 2022).

Brooke shares that you will reap the advantages of your IF lifestyle if you stay within your eating and fasting time frames. Another helpful hint from Brooke is to consume foods rich in good fats, including avocados, olives, nuts, and seeds (note—all plant-based!). These foods are also recognized as brain food and will increase your energy levels and physical strength.

Exercise is a large part of Brooke's life; she works out five days a week, resting on the other two. Brooke suggests that you spend the two days you aren't exercising doing something you enjoy, such as gardening, taking the dog for a walk, or a stroll around the neighborhood. Physical activity awakens chemicals in your brain that essentially relax you and therefore improve your mood. Those chemicals are called endorphins and are transported throughout your body when you exercise. Another benefit of exercising is that it reduces anxiety, lifts your spirits, and gives you self-confidence. When paired with the same benefits of IF, this combo is fantastic.

Brook stresses the importance of including strength training in your routine, especially if you seek a flatter stomach. By doing core exercises, you can also strengthen other areas of your body simultaneously (for instance, planks tone not only your core muscles, but also those of your back, shoulders, and upper arms). An added benefit of strength training is that lean muscle burns more calories; as your muscle mass increases, so will your metabolism. In addition to her workouts, Brooke includes a 45-minute walk in her daily schedule.

INTERMITTENT FASTING AND EXERCISE

It is true that you can do intermittent fasting without exercise and still potentially lose weight. But weight loss is not, as we know, the only reason to make a lifestyle change. The main focus of an IF lifestyle should be to improve overall health and well-being. By adding (or maintaining) exercise while doing IF, you will likely experience added health benefits. Your fitness routine should be individualized to your needs and will depend on things like your age, nutrition intake, lifestyle, overall health status, fitness level, and goals.

The first question people usually ask is, "Is it safe to exercise when fasting?" The short answer is yes. That said, you know your body, and you need to listen to it for any signs of distress, such as feeling weak or lightheaded. Ensure that you are consuming the necessary nutrients and calories during your eating window to sustain yourself without putting strain on your health. If you are feeling fatigue, weakness, or lightheadedness during exercise (or fasting), try adding a pinch of natural sea salt or pink Himalayan salt to your water or coffee. This is a natural way to increase your sodium levels and supplement the electrolytes you are sweating out. Also, remember to keep yourself well-hydrated at all times. When first incorporating exercise into your IF routine, it is advisable to start off easy and gradually build intensity to see what you can tolerate. Also, consult with your care provider if you are new to exercise or in poor physical health.

It is common to struggle during exercise for the first few weeks after transitioning to an intermittent fasting lifestyle, but as your body gets used to the changes, this should resolve. It is used to using your glucose stores for energy, and yours will be depleted from fasting. The upside is that once your body transitions, it will start burning fat for fuel instead, and you will not only feel better but will see maximum rewards for your exercise as a result. If you do not start feeling better after a few weeks, try tweaking your exercise routine or timing to find what works best for you.

Another frequently asked question is regarding the timing of exercise while practicing IF. This is an individual decision you will need to make based on things like your free time and how that corresponds with your eating and fasting windows, but there is evidence that exercising during your fasting window can increase fat burning. The downside of pairing exercise and fasting is that you may find yourself too low-energy to get the most out of your workouts. If this is true, I suggest either moving your exercise closer to the end of your eating window (to include calorie intake closer to your exercise time) or exercising during your eating window. Do what you need to do to make exercise a reality.

Pros and Cons of Exercising While Doing Intermittent Fasting

There are pros and cons to everything, and exercising while doing IF is no exception, though, in my opinion, the pros outweigh the cons. The cons are also usually easy to remedy with just a few minor tweaks in routine. Let's take a look.

Pros

One of the biggest pros to combining exercise and IF is that many people can still lose weight without changing their eating habits. Exercise boosts fat burning, as does fasting, and the combination can melt away the pounds. Studies have shown that people who work out while fasting burn more fat than those who work out after eating a meal.

Combining exercise and fasting has anti-aging effects and can actually slow the aging process. That's definitely good news! The combo also has the potential to boost autophagy, recycling and removing damaged and unwanted cells while creating new, healthier ones. Another benefit is a heightened immune system, which decreases the risk of potential diseases.

Cons

The cons to exercising while doing IF are a shorter list. The most notable are the potential for a drop in blood sugar levels, a sudden drop in blood pressure, and a decrease in performance level due to a lack of adequate fuel to power your body during exercise. The symptoms for all of these include lightheadedness, dizziness, fatigue, or feeling faint. They can usually be remedied by tweaking your exercise routine or moving your exercise times into your eating window. (If these symptoms persist despite making adjustments, consult with your primary care provider).

If you are already an exerciser, continue your current routine and see how it works for you. You may need to adjust your intensity a bit in the beginning as you add in IF, but chances are you will be able to tolerate your routine in no time. If you have never had a regular exercise routine or are struggling during your workouts, start with a low-intensity routine and then try some autotuning to tweak the intensity, timing, or type of exercise until you find something comfortable. Build up from there, as tolerated. Continue evaluating the effects of exercise and your adjustments, and note them in your journal for reference. Never stop challenging yourself, but make sure to listen to your body.

Here is a summary of helpful tips to consider when adding exercise to IF:

- stay hydrated
- ensure that you keep your electrolyte levels up
- keep your fitness routine at a minimum intensity level until you are comfortable ramping up your workout
- choose a fasting plan that works well for you
- consult your medical professional before starting a fitness routine, or change in lifestyle
- *LISTEN TO YOUR BODY!*

Planning Your Exercise

When incorporating exercise into an intermittent fasting lifestyle, planning your exercise and the activities surrounding it is essential. Some things to consider are the types of exercises best suited to IF, what times work best for your workout window, and the foods that will maximize your exercise benefits. Below are some recommendations, but remember—these considerations are like everything else with IF: flexible and amenable to suit your needs.

Types of Exercises

There are two different types of exercises that you can incorporate into your workout routine. One is aerobic exercise (aka "cardio") which is a workout that gets the heart working over a sustained period by doing things like swimming, running, cycling, or walking. The other is anaerobic exercise, for example, strength training or sprinting. This type of exercise pushes you to your maximum limit over a short period of time.

Deciding which types of exercise to do depends on you and your IF schedule. If you are doing daily fasts, such as 16:8 or 18:6, for example, you could do either anaerobic or aerobic exercise or a combination of both. If you are new to intermittent fasting, however, or are following the alternate-day (ADF) method, you may want to either exercise on the days that you are eating or choose low-intensity cardio (aerobic) workouts on the days that you are fasting.

There is some debate about whether you should exercise during your fasting or eating windows, and I have discussed some pros and cons. Ultimately, your choice should depend on how you feel when you are working out. If you are not reaching your desired goals, or performing satisfactorily, try changing your fitness routine or switching your eating or fasting times. Adjust, adjust, and adjust some more until you find what's right for you.

Typical IF Exercise Food

Knowing what to eat and when can go a long way in maximizing your workouts. It is best not to eat immediately before exercise. If you are working out either in your eating window or soon after your fasting window starts, it is essential that you consume a meal that is rich in complex carbohydrates and protein at least two to three hours before you exercise. A good example would be oatmeal with unsweetened soy milk, topped with fresh berries and pumpkin seeds. Or a tofu scramble with onions, peppers, and salsa, with a side of whole grain toast.

After your workout (within your eating window), you should consume healthy carbs, protein, and good fats to aid post-workout recovery. Remember to always focus on whole anti-inflammatory foods which are healing and nutritious, and give your body the fuel it needs to boost your energy levels, increase your metabolism, and keep you happy and healthy.

Adding Supplements to Your Daily Routine

I wholeheartedly believe it is best to get your nutrients from food and not supplements when at all possible. And the fact is that it is possible to get most, if not everything, your body needs from food if you follow an anti-inflammatory, plant-strong diet and eat a large variety of plant foods daily. That said, the restricted eating times and fewer meals associated with intermittent fasting can make it more challenging to eat the same variety that was possible with three meals a day plus snacks. As a result, some people choose to take supplements.

Whether you should take supplements while fasting is entirely up to you and your healthcare provider. If you decide to supplement, it is important to know which should be taken with food and which should be taken on an empty stomach so that you can plan to take them during your eating or fasting window appropriately. The following should be taken with food during your eating window:

- magnesium
- zinc or copper
- turmeric or curcumin
- omega krill complex or krill oil
- vitamins A, D, and K, which are fat-soluble
- amino acids or combinations
- omega-3 fatty acids or medium-chain triglycerides (MTCs)
- protein powders
- electrolyte powders or effervescent tablets that are sweetened
- sweetened chewable supplements and gummies
- supplements made with cane sugar, fruit juice, or starches, including sweeteners

These supplements should be taken on an empty stomach and can be taken during your fasting window:

- iron
- folic acid
- probiotics
- tyrosine
- vitamins B and C, which are water-soluble

Plant-Based Diet and Supplements

If switching to a plant-based diet, there are some important nutrients you will likely need to supplement, as they are only found in animal foods or fortified, processed foods. These are:

- vitamin B12
- vitamin D
- omega-3
- iodine
- calcium
- zinc
- iron- is absorbed best on an empty stomach but may cause significant stomach upset. Always take it with a full glass of water. Move to your eating window if stomach upset persists.

A well-rounded vegan multivitamin, such as Dr. Fuhrman's Women's Daily Multivitamin +D3, is a good way to get most or all of your needed supplements in one source.

It is important to note that many meat-eaters are also deficient in these nutrients. A plant-based diet, despite sometimes needing supplementation, is still arguably the healthiest way to eat.

*Just a reminder to consult your healthcare provider before adding any supplements to your daily routine. Be sure to request blood tests to determine what your body actually requires.

9

A HAPPY MEAL—PROPER PLANNING AND PREPARATION

I want this chapter to serve as a simple guide to help you plan and prepare your meals without being over-whelmed. Sometimes, transitioning to the IF lifestyle is a little daunting. In the beginning, you will find yourself watching the time and obsessing about what you will eat. Eventually, however, you will find that intermittent fasting takes less time, thought, and preparation than a standard eating method. The tips in this chapter will help. But first, let's look at some fun facts about food, eating, and weight loss.

One study found that if your workstation is disorganized, you may turn to unhealthy snacks. People who have bowls of candy on their desks also report weighing 15.4 pounds more than those who don't.

Eating off red plates helps individuals eat less, possibly because red is the color of caution, danger, and a warning to stop.

Using cash instead of credit cards or digital payment causes people to purchase healthier food.

Turning down the temperature in your bedroom may be beneficial to your weight loss, as research has shown that people sleeping in cold rooms burn 7% more calories overnight than those in a warm room.

Smelling peppermint on a regular basis decreases both appetite and calorie intake[1] (Lenhardt, 2017).

THE ART OF MEAL PLANNING

I believe that meal planning is essential in every home and is something that we all should be doing. We spend so much money on fast food, convenience meals, and unhealthy calorie-dense snacks that we are putting our health at risk—not to mention our finances. A common argument is that people don't have time to cook healthy meals after a long day at work, and the family is chomping at the bit to eat. At that point, without proper planning, it is easier just to grab meals from the drive-through, order delivery, or heat up something from a box in the freezer. At this point, you've lost the battle before it's begun.

Planning your meals with intention will ensure that everyone is fed on time and will eat healthy, delicious meals that fuel their bodies and satisfy their hunger. It will also prevent making poor choices when your fasting window ends and you're starving without any food in the house. Meal planning doesn't have to be complicated or time-consuming. Pick a day and time each week (maybe your Saturday morning coffee time?) and grab your food journal. Take a few minutes to plan out your meals for the week ahead. That's it! This brief time at the beginning of your week will save you hours of indecision and frustration later on.

In addition to your journal, you can use a calorie guide or app to help plan your meals and ensure that you get adequate nutrition during your eating window. I have also included a sample weekly meal plan in the next section to use as a template and give you ideas for how to arrange your meals. Lastly, take advantage of the recipes in the back of this book or the many plant-based cooking sites on the internet for inspiration for delicious, healthy meals. I will include some of my favorites at the end of the chapter.

Instead of being a burden, meal planning will lighten your load and ultimately give you more time to focus on reaching your goals. One of the bonuses of IF is that you will be eating fewer meals, which frees up time that used to be spent planning and preparing those meals. Meal planning takes the guesswork out of dinnertime. It will also save you money in the long run, as you will be cooking healthy, fresh meals at home rather than eating out or calling for delivery. Switching to a more plant-focused diet will save you money, as fresh fruit, vegetables, whole grains, and legumes are much cheaper than meat, dairy, and processed foods. I suggest that you treat yourself by using those savings for a manicure, pedicure, facial, massage, or spa treatment. You're worth it!

Helpful Tips for Meal Planning

Here are some tips for successful meal planning:

- As a beginner to the IF lifestyle, start small. Begin by planning for a few days at a time, or a week maximum, to get the feel for meal planning and see what works for you.
- Remember to incorporate ingredients from each food group (healthy fats, carbs, and protein) into your meals to ensure that you get all the nutrients your body requires.
- Build a menu around your ingredient choices above.
- Ensure that you have the necessary ingredients for your meals in the pantry, freezer, and refrigerator (and move snacks to a place where they are "out of sight and out of mind").
- Never go grocery shopping when you are hungry, and work off a list of needed ingredients rather than browsing the aisles at the grocery store.

- Avoid recipes with special ingredients you will not frequently use or substitute things you have on hand.
- Stock up on multi-purpose foods such as quinoa, spinach, or buckwheat, which you could turn into fresh salads for those hot summer days or delicious hearty soups for the winter months.
- Break the monotony of your meals—which could cause boredom and overeating. Search for seasonal recipes, or be creative and add your own flair to classic recipes.
- Make extra food to freeze or store it in the refrigerator for meals later in the week.
- Think ahead, and incorporate your leftovers into the meals you will prepare for the next few days.

TAKING MEAL PLANNING TO THE PREPPING STAGE

Where meal planning is setting up a menu and planning meals for the days ahead, meal prepping is preparing the full meals or components of that menu and portioning them out as grab-and-go meals so that you can have dinner on the table in minutes. You can put containers of meals in the fridge to eat before a workout, have snacks ready to grab once your eating window opens, or put meals in the freezer for use on another night. If done right, meal planning and prepping can take all of the pressure off of deciding what to eat. It will already be decided for you, and you can spend that time and energy on something else.

Besides offering a variety of meal options to eat during your feasting window, meal planning and prepping cuts down on cost and food waste by intentionally using the foods you buy and utilizing leftovers as meals for another day. It allows you to be intentional about the foods you are putting in your body and helps ensure that you get the nutrients you need to fuel it. It also goes a long way toward helping you make good food choices when hungry, as there will always be something ready-to-eat in your fridge or freezer.

Helpful Tips for Meal Prepping

- Select a meal prep method that best fits your lifestyle and nutritional needs.
- Choose user-friendly, easy recipes when first learning meal prep.
- Make sure to have meals and snacks ready to go when your eating window hits. An empty stomach and an empty fridge are a recipe for disaster!
- Prepare some of your favorite (healthy) comfort foods to add enjoyment to your meals.
- Prepare enough food to store in airtight containers or freezer bags, to use as meals later in the week.
- Keep a variety of vegetables pre-cut in containers to eat as snacks (with salsa, hummus, or other dips), or

use them in your salads, soups, stir-fries, or buddha bowls.

- Stock up on healthy, whole-food snacks, and keep them where you will see them when you open the refrigerator, pantry, or drawer—this will minimize your cravings for unhealthy snacks.
- Keep cubed or diced fresh fruit in your freezer or refrigerator for a quick smoothie or yogurt topping.
- Keep a variety of cooked beans, tofu, and whole grains in containers in your fridge or freezer to make a quick meal. These are good in salads, soups, stews, or "bowls." Can also be incorporated into wraps or burritos for an impromptu meal change.

I dedicate one day a week to planning and prepping all of my meals. I have a hectic, long work schedule, and if I have my meals ready in advance, I make good food choices when my eating window hits. I also run the risk of binge eating, and I don't want to go there. Having healthy, delicious meals waiting for me when I get home helps to keep me on track and helps me know what I am putting into my body in terms of calories, nutrients, and portion sizes. It also frees up that time that would normally be spent cooking for something more interesting.

Now that we've explained meal planning and prepping, we can move on to perhaps the most important part—choosing what to eat. In the next chapter, I will give some recommendations to help you get started.

10

EAT THIS AND THAT—ANTI-INFLAMMATORY OR BUST!

When switching to an anti-inflammatory or plant-based way of eating, you want to ensure that your diet includes adequate protein, carbohydrates, fiber, and healthy fats. The good news is that plant foods provide a large variety of each of these (in fact, plant foods are the only foods that contain fiber), and if you are eating well-rounded meals, the plant-based anti-inflammatory diet should give you all you need. With this way of eating, it is not necessary to count macros or calculate percentages—unless, of course, you have an underlying medical condition and your health provider or dietician has recommended it. By "eating the rainbow," you will fuel your body with pure, clean nutrition and get much-needed antioxidants for healing and restoration.

KEY COMPONENTS

So far, we've taken a good look at both intermittent fasting and the benefits to optimal weight management and overall health and well-being. We've talked about different IF plans and how to choose one that's right for your lifestyle. We've also touched on the anti-inflammatory diet component and the added benefits of going plant-based, but this is where I'd like to dive a little deeper. Our bodies need a wide array of vitamins, minerals, and macronutrients to run at maximum efficiency and capacity. By ensuring that we are incorporating foods from every beneficial food group, we can ensure that our body gets the nutrition it needs (and deserves).

A Closer Look at the Food Groups

First of all, what are the food groups? Regardless of your eating style, the food groups are fruits, vegetables, grains, protein foods, dairy, and fats. What you eat within these food groups varies depending on your diet of choice. With the plant-based anti-inflammatory lifestyle, we will focus on getting all our nutrients from plant sources. I am often asked if it is possible to get everything we need while eating this way. "How do you get enough protein?" is probably the most common question. I want to assure you that if you eat enough calories to sustain your body on a plant-based diet, you will consume enough protein. All plant foods contain protein. Consider the biggest, strongest animals on the planet—gorillas, rhinoceros, hippopotami, horses, and elephants. Every one of them eats a 100% plant-based diet. If they can get enough of what they need from plants, so can we.

Let's take a look at what falls into each plant-based food group, and I will also provide a sample shopping list for each so that you can have plenty of healthy, delicious plant-based foods available for your meals and snacks.

Protein Foods

Legumes

Legumes include beans, peas, and lentils. They are an excellent source of protein and fiber. Legumes are cholesterol-free, low in fat, and packed with nutrients. The fat they do contain is a healthy fat. They are versatile and can be consumed in soups, salads, stews, or buddha bowls. The options are endless. A can of chickpeas blended with garlic, salt, pepper, and a splash of lemon juice makes a healthy and delicious dip for your freshly cut vegetables or can be used as a salad dressing.

Your shopping list:

- chickpeas
- kidney beans
- lentils
- lima beans
- black beans
- raw peanuts

- pinto beans
- split peas
- black-eyed peas
- white beans
- fava beans
- mung beans
- popcorn
- string beans

Soy

Soy is an all-star in the plant-based community because it is high in protein and a natural source of healthy fats, vitamins, and minerals. The early belief was that soy products increased the risk of breast cancer, but that has been dispelled. Moderate amounts of soy are not only safe but may decrease the risk of some cancers. The next time you shop at your local Whole Foods store, don't hesitate to add a couple of soy-based products to your cart.

Your shopping list:

- tofu
- tempeh
- edamame
- miso–which adds flavor to your soups and stews

Healthy Fats

Nuts and Seeds

Nuts and seeds, like many other plant foods, cross categories. They are comprised of healthy fats and also provide protein, vitamins, and minerals. Remember to buy raw, unseasoned, and unsalted nuts. While roasted nuts still contain good nutrition, raw nuts are healthier. Roasting may destroy some of the nutrients and antioxidants in nuts, and the high temperatures used for roasting can oxidize the fat and create a toxic compound called acrylamide. All that aside, the added oil, salt, and seasoning in roasted nuts can not only increase calories but can also trigger us to eat more. Remember that nuts and seeds are naturally high-calorie foods, even in their raw form, so eat sparingly and pay attention to portion sizes.

Try nuts and seeds sprinkled on oatmeal, in granola, or enjoy as salad or soup toppers.

Your shopping list:

- nut butter—choose a natural variety to avoid oil, sugar, or other additives
- almonds
- pecans
- pumpkin seeds
- Brazil nuts
- flaxseed

- sesame seeds
- chia seeds
- cashews
- macadamia nuts
- sunflower seeds
- walnuts
- hemp seeds
- tahini—sauce made of ground sesame seeds (This is a key ingredient in hummus and can also be used to make salad dressing or dip)
- pine nuts

Carbohydrates

Whole Grains

Whole grains are high-fiber foods that also provide protein, vitamins, and minerals to your diet. They are complex carbohydrates, and women over 50 should eat 6–7 servings daily. Their fiber content will keep you full longer and give you a greater sense of satiety after eating. The benefits of eating whole grains are lower cholesterol, as well as lower risk of cancer, heart disease, type II diabetes, and other illnesses.

*Note that gluten can cause inflammation in some people. Avoid wheat, rye, barley, spelt, and malt if you are sensitive to gluten.

Your shopping list:

- barley—contains gluten
- buckwheat—despite the name, there is no "wheat" in buckwheat; it is classified as a whole grain but is actually a type of seed
- cornmeal
- wheat or whole wheat pasta—contains gluten
- oats—considered the most nutritious grain
- quinoa—is classified as a grain but is technically a seed; one of the most nutritious grains
- brown rice
- millet
- rye—contains gluten
- spelt—contains gluten
- sorghum
- amaranth

Dairy Alternatives

Many of us were raised on dairy products, so doing away with milk, yogurt, and cheese may be a little daunting. It is important to know that as we age, it is common to experience problems with our gut health, and lactose intolerance is often the culprit. Dairy is also inflammatory in other ways, and the protein in milk (casein) has been found to cause cancer in animal studies. You can still enjoy your dairy—switch to milk, cheese, or yogurt that has been made with plant-based milk, as well as vitamin B12 and/or vitamin D fortified. If buying dairy alternatives, particularly cheese, it is essential to read the labels. Many of them are made primarily from oils and other unhealthy ingredients and may set you back in your health and weight-loss goals if you consume too much.

Your shopping list:

- milk—almond, oat, cashew, soy, macadamia, hemp seed, etc... Coconut milk is high in calories and saturated fat and is best used sparingly in cooking rather than as a beverage.
- plant-based yogurt—plain, unsweetened varieties are the healthiest. Read the labels. For fruit-flavored yogurt, make your own at home by blending unsweetened yogurt with fresh berries and a touch of maple syrup or honey.
- non-dairy cheese—look for nut-based varieties rather than oil-based for the most health benefits. These alternatives are best used sparingly and occasionally. They tend to be high in calories and low in nutritional value.

Fruits and Vegetables

These are my favorite food groups. They come in an endless variety, can usually be eaten either cooked or raw, are simple to prepare, and are always available in some form, whether raw, frozen, or canned. If possible, stick to fresh or frozen for maximum freshness and nutritional value, as well as no additives. The current dietary guidelines say that women over 50 should eat approximately 1 1/2 cups of fruit and 2 cups of vegetables daily. That should be seen as a minimum and not a maximum. On a plant-based diet, you may eat unlimited fresh, whole fruits and veggies and eat until you are satisfied. If you are focused on weight loss, however, it may be beneficial to limit fruit and stick to less starchy vegetables, which have fewer calories. All fruits and vegetables have excellent health benefits, and none are "off limits" in an anti-inflammatory lifestyle.

Your shopping list:

Vegetables:

- asparagus
- broccoli
- cabbage
- brussels sprouts
- artichoke hearts
- celery
- cucumber
- mushrooms
- onions
- eggplant

- carrots
- peppers
- cauliflower
- radish
- zucchini
- bok choy
- arugula
- kale
- swiss chard
- spinach
- collard greens
- romaine
- butternut squash
- corn
- yam
- parsnips
- beets
- pumpkin
- potatoes

Fruits:

- avocados— can technically fit under fruit, vegetables, or healthy fats. They are loaded with nutrients but also loaded with calories and fat. Eat sparingly and pay attention to portion size if you are trying to lose weight.

- bananas
- figs
- grapes
- jackfruit
- plums
- pineapples
- cherries
- apples
- watermelon
- pears
- mango
- peaches
- grapefruit
- lime
- oranges
- lemons
- tangerines
- raspberries
- blueberries
- strawberries
- blackberries

When making your shopping list, you can either make your meal plan and then make your shopping list based on the meals you plan to prepare, or you can shop and create your meals from the foods you purchased. If you choose to do the latter, it can help to think about filling your cart with

- nutrient-dense foods such as leafy greens and colorful fruits and vegetables. Both fresh or frozen are great, and canned will work in a pinch, but make sure to read those labels for hidden ingredients such as sugar or oil. Also, watch the sodium content of canned foods.
- high-fiber foods such as whole grains, flax seed, fruits and vegetables.
- unrefined carbohydrates/starches such as potato, sweet potato, brown rice, oats, and quinoa.
- foods that are low in added sugar, sodium, and fat (minimize processed foods).
- some sources of healthy fats such as avocado, nuts, and seeds.
- enough food to cover your nutrient and caloric needs.
- some sources of protein, such as nuts, seeds, lentils, beans, tofu, tempeh, and edamame.

It is also helpful to have a good supply of herbs and spices on hand, to add flavor to your meals. Vegetable stock is a must-have for sautéing and making soups. As an alternative to purchasing it, you can use your vegetable scraps and peels to make your own. Just store scraps in the freezer until you have a full batch—then boil for an hour and strain to extract the broth. Another plant-based staple is nutritional yeast, which adds a savory "cheesy" flavor to dishes and is a good source of protein, and B12 if you purchase the fortified variety.

Now that we have the basic food knowledge, it is time to plan your menu and prep your meals. I have included a sample menu, but please feel free to substitute in the meals that sound good to you and your family. Also, remember to utilize leftovers to make life easier, and reduce the number of meals you need to cook. Please note that since we are intermittent fasting, we will not be eating three meals a day (unless you are doing a 5:2, ADF, or another method that allows for full days of food). I am including them just so that you can have a wide variety of meals to choose from. I also found it hard at first to get in all of my needed nutrition because I used to eat oats with fruit every morning, and when I switched to eating only lunch and dinner, my oatmeal went out the window. I have since started eating "breakfast for dinner" or having banana oat pancakes for a snack once or twice a week. Use your creativity, and you can make this work for you, too!

YOUR VERY OWN SAMPLE MENU

Monday	Overnight Oats With Apple, Cinnamon, Walnuts. Glass of Plant Milk	Vegetable Hummus Wraps (Whole Grain)	Southwest Stuffed Bell Peppers (Brown Rice, Veggies, Topped With Salsa)
Tuesday	Avocado Whole Grain Toast Topped With Sliced Onion and Tomato	Black Bean and Southwest Veggie Bowl	Lentil Shepherd's Pie
Wednesday	Southwest Tofu Scramble (With Onions, Pepper, and Black Olives) Topped With Salsa	Minestrone Bean Soup, Side Salad With Tahini Dressing	Chickpea Meatloaf and Roasted Potatoes
Thursday	Smoothie With Frozen Bananas, Greens, Chia Seeds, and Plant Milk	Vegetable Pho Soup, Fresh Veggie Summer Rolls	Vegetarian Black Bean Chili (Leftovers Black Beans and Veggies From Bowl)
Friday	Oatmeal With Wild Blueberries, Pumpkin Seeds, Plant Milk and Nut Butter (or Make Double Batch of Overnight Oats on Monday and Eat Leftovers Here)	Chickpea Meatloaf Sandwich (Leftovers), Veggies and Salsa	Lentil Shepherd's Pie Leftovers
Saturday	Fresh Fruit Bowl, Whole Grain Toast Topped With Nut Butter	Southwest Stuffed Bell Peppers (Leftovers)	White Bean Meatballs With Spaghetti, Sautéed Kale
Sunday	Banana Oat Pancakes Topped With Fresh Blueberries and Strawberries	Veggie Salad With Hummus Dressing	Chili (Leftover) With Corn Tortillas and Guacamole

Here are a few of my favorite sites for plant-based recipes.

• www.forksoverknives.com —this site is great for articles and tips on getting started on a whole food plant-based (WFPB) way of eating, as well as delicious recipes.

- shaneandsimple.com

- minimalistbaker.com

- monkeyandmekitchenadventures.com

- www.pickuplimes.com

- www.karissasvegankitchen.com

I have included 50 simple plant-based recipes at the back of this book to get you started. Bon appétit!

MY PHYSICAL ABILITY BEFORE AND AFTER STARTING AN ANTI-INFLAMMATORY IF LIFESTYLE

I am a doer. I have always had what I call "the soul of an athlete," though I have never been very athletic. My heart and mind were willing, but my flesh was weak, so to speak. Had I known I was struggling with a lifelong disorder that affected both my arms and legs, I may have given up (I guess there can be blessing in ignorance, after all!), but since I thought I was perfectly healthy, I kept trying. I would say to myself, "If he/she can do it, so can I." I did not allow myself any excuses. Now, that's NOT to say that I was good at all those things I tried to do. When it came to physical activity, I was actually pretty dreadful. I was slow and uncoordinated. I was literally the last to finish any race in school and finished solidly with the back of the pack in all of the public races I entered (with the 5-year-old girl and the 80-year-old man with the tiny dog on a leash). I played basketball because I was 6 feet tall by the time I finished 6th grade, and still managed to be bad at it. I couldn't get down the court fast enough. I have tried nearly every sport, outdoor activity, and gym routine. I thought if I tried hard enough, I would eventually and miraculously be good enough. I never really was, but I also never quit.

As I was nearing 50, I decided that I needed to do one last big feat to prove that I still could. Fifty was hard for me, and I was trying desperately to hold on to what was left of my youth and my dignity. My friend and "travel wife" Mandy (21 years younger than me) and I decided to climb Mt. Kilimanjaro in Tanzania. Well, I decided on it by pure whim, and she is always game for any good adventure I dream up. So it was set. One month before my 50th birthday, we met in Africa, and on March 24, 2018, we started our trek. It was seven days of bliss and two days of hell.

March 30, summit day, was 17 hours long and included 4,000 feet of elevation gain straight up to the summit (19, 341 feet) and then another 6,000 feet of elevation straight down to our camp that night. I have never been so tested or tired in my entire life. "I can take one more step" became the mantra we used to keep going. Just one more step. About halfway down from the summit, my legs stopped working properly. They grew increasingly heavy and immobile. I couldn't bend them fully at the knees and was left swinging them from the hip for each forward step. I couldn't lift my feet fully off the ground and was dragging them across the rocky surface of the riverbed we were walking. I fell behind with my guide as the others powered on ahead. It had begun to rain and became cold, slippery, and much harder to move as time went on. With every fiber of my being, I wanted to be back at camp—but no matter what I tried, it was no use. I couldn't go any faster. I reached camp after dark, several hours after Mandy and her guide had arrived. I had prevailed —we had reached the summit of Mt. Kilimanjaro, proving I "still could," but I wasn't okay. I was not only suffering the debilitating effects of what I would later find out was Lipedema, but I also had pneumonia and a bleed in my lower GI tract. I was beginning to wonder if I would ever be able to do these things again, or if life ended at 50.

This is not to focus on the negative. First of all, I summited Mt. Kilimanjaro—the highest point in Africa and the highest free-standing mountain in the world! And I did it six weeks shy of my 50th birthday! But I was far from healthy. That needed to change. Enter the anti-inflammatory, intermittent fasting lifestyle that I adopted less than a year later in an attempt to get my life back on track. It not only helped me lose weight but also greatly improved my health and mobility despite my Lipedema. I want to fast forward four years to May 10th, 2022—the day after my 54th birthday. That is the day I left with my cousins to trek to Mt. Everest Base Camp in Nepal. That soul of an athlete never did leave me, and I was giving it another shot! I had been sick in the weeks that preceded the trek and was also recuperating from a back injury from a fall down a mountain path about two months prior. All of the insecurities and questions began arising again. Despite how much better I felt at this stage in my life, I wondered if I was past the point where I should be doing this. The trek was no joke—10 days, reaching an altitude of 17,585 feet, with a summit of Kala Patthar mountain (18,519 feet) the next morning.

Friends told me that it was impossible to do both Base Camp and Kala Patthar on the same trip and that I needed to choose which victory to shoot for. I knew, however, that others had completed both, and I still stood by the adage, "If he/she can do it, so can I!" I knew I had to try. I won't give the details, but I felt amazing on that trek. Like a beast. All the other members of the trip struggled with either illness or altitude sickness at some point during those 10 days, but I never did. I felt strong. My legs kept moving. They didn't swell or become heavy. My breathing was solid. I didn't get sick. I felt like a million bucks. I also managed to do that Kala Patthar summit. I won't pretend that was easy, but I made it. Only one other person on our five-member team, the 50-year-old son-in-law of one of my cousins, even attempted it. He made it as well. I know, without a doubt, that my success on that trip can be 100% attributed to my way of eating and the lifestyle changes I had made in the previous 3 ½ years. Life didn't end at 50. For me, it began again.

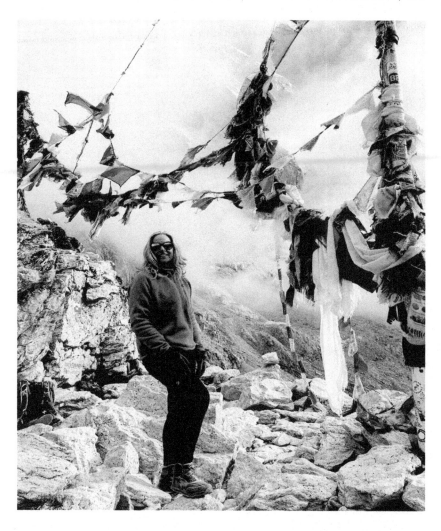

The author, age 54, on the summit of Kala Patthar mountain in Nepal (elevation 18,519 feet) the morning after reaching Mt. Everest base camp (17,598 feet).

11

THE LAST MILE—FINAL FACTORS FOR IF SUCCESS

We're almost there! We've covered the IF basics, methods, benefits, and information to help you switch to an anti-inflammatory eating lifestyle. What more could you need? Maybe just a few final tips to ensure your success. Switching to and sticking to a new lifestyle can be daunting, but there are ways to make this one a little bit easier.

TIPS AND TRICKS

Below are some things that I found useful as I embarked on my IF journey. I hope you will find them helpful, too, as you move forward. Please feel free to use the ones that work for you and disregard the ones that don't, and remember—this is your lifestyle.

Socializing

How to keep your social life while on IF—you can still reap the benefits of intermittent fasting without sacrificing your social life. The key is to be flexible and schedule your eating periods around when you need to go out with friends and family.

- **Socializing in the morning**—if your eating window isn't in the morning, try meeting friends at a time that doesn't fall during normal breakfast times, and instead, meet for a cup of (black) coffee or a walk!
- **Socializing mid-day**—if you are doing intermittent fasting daily, and your eating window spans both lunch and dinner, it is often possible to meet people for lunch. Try to schedule your timing so that by the time your food arrives, so has your window. For instance, if your eating window is from 1 p.m.–7 p.m. daily, then try to meet no earlier than 12:30 p.m. so that it will be 1 pm or close to it by the time your meal arrives at the table. If this is not possible and you need to meet earlier, you have a decision to make. Either adjust your eating and fasting windows for the day (remember—it's not the end of the world) or say you've just eaten before arriving and instead enjoy a nice glass of unsweetened iced tea instead of a meal.
- **Socializing at night**–the most common fasting methods involve eating meals in the evening, so this

is perhaps easier to work around than socializing at other times of the day. Remember, though, not to eat until your eating window has started, and make sure to stop by the time it ends. If your dinner is on the late side, this may mean forgoing dessert or not having drinks for the latter part of your event. If you are meeting later in the evening or at night, switch to sparkling water over ice, with a wedge of lime on the edge of the glass only. Don't squeeze it in for a clean fast!

- **Socializing without food**—this can be tricky, as so much of our socialization and celebrations involve eating and drinking. If possible, be creative and meet with friends for something that doesn't include food. Go for a walk, attend a seminar or class together, go bowling, or browse a bookstore. If you want to sit down for a "chew and chat," opt for a cafe during non-meal times and have a cup of coffee or tea. If others are pressuring you to eat (and this will happen), you have a choice to make. You can lie (I am only kind of kidding here) and tell them that you have a doctor's appointment or lab work in the morning and you have to be fasting for it, or just tell them the truth. Share your story with them, explain that you are doing IF for your health, and invite them to join you!

Your Fasting Window

The most important thing is the fasting window. That is when your body is reaping the maximum benefits of this lifestyle. The length of your eating window is less crucial, though it may alter the number of calories you are ingesting, so be conscious of that and adjust according to your daily needs. To make this way of life user-friendly, move your fasting times as needed to allow yourself the most flexibility to enjoy time with family and friends. For instance, if you choose to do 18:6 fasting, you might opt to make your eating window from 12 p.m.–6 p.m. or 1 p.m.–7 p.m. to allow for both lunch and dinner at "normal" meal times. And remember not to obsess over the numbers. You don't have to be exact and perfect every day. If you are eating out with family and friends and your dinner lasts until 7:30 p.m., don't stress. Consider fasting until 1:30 p.m. the next day and shortening your eating window to get back on track. Or don't! Tomorrow is a new day, and the benefits of this life-style are cumulative. One off-day (or even a few) won't derail all the good you've done. Just start again.

As I write this, it is 7 p.m., and I am eating a bean burrito bowl. My fasting window starts at 5:30 p.m. I had a long day, and my fridge was empty. By the time I had dinner ready, it was 6:30 p.m. It happens. Life happens.

Remember that this is a lifestyle, not a diet, so commit to the long haul, and you will see results. The best way of eating is one you will stick to; a bit of flexibility will help with that!

Tracking Your Progress

Keeping track of your progress can help motivate you to continue. It can also bring your attention to mistakes or plateaus in your progress.

- **Weigh yourself**: But don't weigh daily. Weight can fluctuate for many reasons (including stressing about weight!), and the general trend is more important than the daily numbers. It also takes time for the body to deplete glycogen stores, start burning fat for fuel, and let go of those unwanted pounds. I would suggest weighing no more than every couple of weeks in the beginning and definitely not more than weekly. Once you have a good handle on this lifestyle and what you need in terms of food, calories, eating and fasting windows, I would suggest weighing monthly or less (or not at all!) and focusing on how your body looks and feels as a gauge to how you're doing.
- **Measure inches**: (either manually using a tape measure or using apps like MeThreeSixty to do digital scans/measurements). With IF, your body composition will often change, even if your weight does not. Measurements can be a better reflection of what is going on in your body than the scale. It is also good to note that lean muscle mass weighs more than the same amount/mass of fat tissue—so your body could remain at the same weight or even more

as you gain lean muscle and lose fat—even if your body stays the same size.

- **Get regular check-ups and lab work**: to measure health progress, like cholesterol levels, blood sugar, blood pressure, etc... Keep in mind that if you are losing weight, your cholesterol levels may be temporarily elevated as your body breaks down fat and releases it into your bloodstream. Once your rapid weight loss slows or stops, your cholesterol levels should normalize/become more accurate.

- **Keep a food journal**: Of what you are eating, how much you are eating, how you feel when you are eating, triggers that caused you to overeat, and things that derail either your fasting window or your eating patterns. Many of us are emotional eaters, and it can be helpful to write our food habits out to help identify what affects us. It can also be beneficial to have a record of what you are eating and how much in the event that you are not losing weight or you are having unintended health effects. Sharing your food diary with a dietician can help make tweaks and changes in your diet to counteract those things.

- **Measure and celebrate non-scale victories**: like fitting into those jeans that didn't fit last month or the ability to run longer or farther than you could last year. Maybe you are sleeping through the night or have mountains of energy during the day! Do you feel sexy and have an increased sex drive? Maybe more confidence? Those things are all indicators that IF is working for you and have nothing to do with a number on a scale.

Finding Support

It is much easier to stick with a healthy regimen when you have support from people who are experiencing and doing the same thing. This can be support from people you know or people you don't, and can be in-person or online. Customize this to work for you and your comfort level. I personally like the ease and accessibility of Facebook groups. Below are some resources; you will find many others on Facebook and the internet. There is literally something for everyone! I personally like the support in intermittent fasting for women over 50 groups.

- www.facebook.com/groups/3033442840221840
- 3fatchicks.com
- www.thecreativefeast.com/intermittent-fasting
- www.reddit.com/r/intermittentfasting/comments/lyeqea/support_group_for_women_fasting/
- www.fitwithrachel.com/intermittent-fasting-support-group/

If you are interested in joining a fabulous group of women for life support in general (not IF specific), please check out my Fit, Fierce, and Fabulous (Women) Over 50 group on FB. We'd love to have you!

- www.facebook.com/groups/
fitfierceandfabulouswomenover50

Over the years, the popularity of intermittent fasting has skyrocketed, thanks to celebrities who swear by it and its fairly easy methods. Unlike diets, IF is a lifestyle strategy not only to achieve your goal weight but your overall health goals as well. Skeptics may say it's not for everyone—but the only way to find out is to try it. If you're looking to shed pounds and improve your overall health and well-being, IF is definitely something to consider.

THE END OF THE JOURNEY

You've made it to the final stretch! Congratulations. I hope this has been an exciting journey for you, filled with stories, facts, research, tips, tools, and information that will be useful to help you find your way to fit, fierce, and fabulous. I am confident that you will now be able to choose the right method for you and successfully reach your goals. There is nothing to lose by giving IF a try but everything to gain. You've got this!

SHARE THE SECRET WITH SOMEONE ELSE!

Now that you know all you need to make a real success of intermittent fasting and embrace being over 50 for all it can offer, you're in a perfect position to help someone else.

Simply by leaving your honest opinion of this book on Amazon, you'll show new readers where they can find the guidance they need to reap the benefits of intermittent fasting and enter the next phase of their life healthier and happier than ever before.

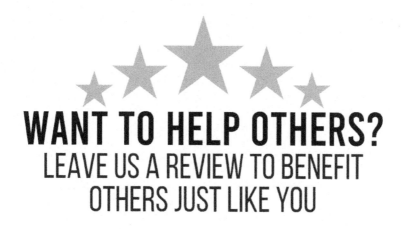

WANT TO HELP OTHERS?
LEAVE US A REVIEW TO BENEFIT OTHERS JUST LIKE YOU

Thank you for your support. All our lives, we are sent a strong message that everything goes downhill after 50... but it really doesn't have to be this way- and together, we can make sure more people know it.

Scan the QR code below for a quick review!

CONCLUSION

Let's recap what we've learned. In the first couple of chapters, we discussed who shouldn't participate in intermittent fasting and looked at disordered eating in detail. Please remember to discontinue IF and seek help if you find it triggering to you in any way. We then discussed and debunked the myths about intermittent fasting and replaced them with solid information.

Chapter 3 took us to intermittent fasting basics, benefits, and possible side effects. We also learned more about why and how IF works in the body. Chapter 4 was a detailed introduction to 10 different methods of practicing IF and the upsides and downsides of each to help you pick a method that best fits your lifestyle and goals. We also discussed the importance of clean fasting to ensure that your body stays in the fasting mode and autophagy during your entire fasting window. We have discussed gender differences and the effects of intermittent fasting on both. In my opinion, the most important chapter of all is Chapter 6, which discusses what to expect in our 50s, including both regular aging changes and potential diseases, and how intermittent fasting can help with each.

We not only discussed intermittent fasting but also whether or not to incorporate exercise, the best exercises to do during intermittent fasting, and tips for safe exercise during the fasting window. We talked about medication use during fasting, what supplements (if using) should be taken with food, and which can be taken during your fasting window.

Not only have we covered fasting, exercise, and supplement use, but we have also learned about the anti-inflammatory diet and the benefits of eating this way. We did a deep dive into plant-based nutrition and how this way of eating can heal your body, such as reducing inflammation, lowering cholesterol, decreasing the risk for disease, and many more. It will also give you more energy, youthfulness, and confidence.

In terms of tips and tricks to make a successful transition to an anti-inflammatory intermittent fasting lifestyle, we have covered meal planning, meal prepping, and shopping for healthy plant-based foods. I have given you a shopping list, a sample weekly meal plan, 50 plant-based recipes, and online resources to get you started.

Lastly, you will find a listing of non-food elements to keep you on track with your IF journey. You have received recommendations for how to track your progress, stay on track while socializing, and find support. I have given you some suggestions for online resources, but please feel free to search for others that meet your individual needs. There is something out there for everyone!

Being "over 50" is better than I ever imagined. As a matter of fact, I imagined that it would be awful. Instead, I have been living my best life for the past few years. I am an IF success story. The longer I do this, the better I feel. When people see photos, they often joke that I am aging backward. The truth is, I feel like I am. I look back at photos from 5 or 10 years ago and look younger and healthier now. I *feel* younger and healthier now. I can't wait to see what 60 brings! Remember —there is no special reason that this worked for me. The fact is that intermittent fasting works. It can work for you, too! All you have to do is make the decision to give it a try. Remember our 30-day challenge? Why not make today "Day One"?

IT'S NOW OR NEVER

I wish I had this book when I started my IF journey. Instead, I had to figure it out on my own. By equipping you with all the tools you need in one place, you can take the opportunity to make the necessary changes and see the results you have always desired! Make the decision today to start on a healing path—body, mind, and spirit—and become the best you, yet!

If you would like more tips on transitioning to a plant-based way of eating, please take a look at my other book, *Plant-Based Basics: An Easy to Follow, Step by Step Guide to Transitioning to a Plant Strong Diet and Lifestyle*, on Amazon.

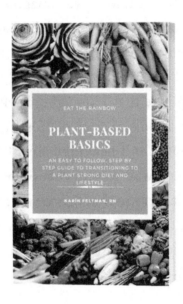

The End

All right—you have everything you need, and I am confident you will successfully reach your goals. Until we meet again, remember to love yourself, give yourself grace, and never stop striving to be Fit, Fierce, and Fabulous Over 50!

If you found this book helpful, help me create a change in someone else's life, too. Please take a couple of minutes to leave a review. Thank you!

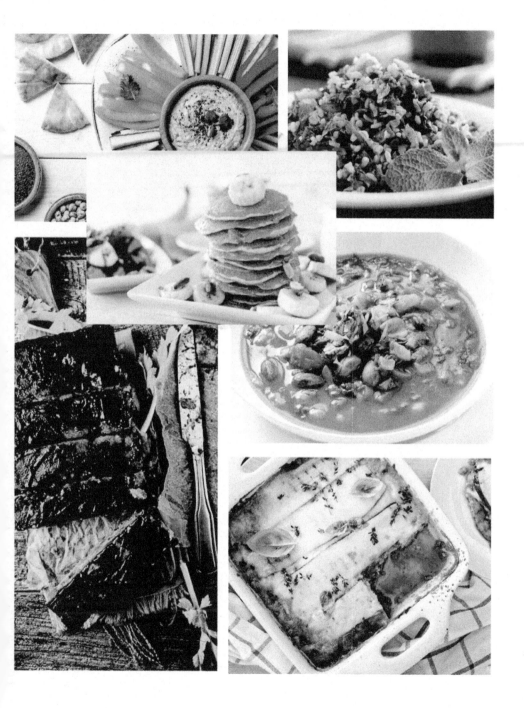

RECIPES—50 PLANT-BASED BASICS TO GET YOU STARTED

The internet is brimming with amazing plant-based recipes, and vegan cookbooks are available in every bookstore. That should make it easier than ever to make the switch to a more plant-strong lifestyle. That said, I think the recent surge in information and availability of resources can be overwhelming. It is hard to know where to start. That is what this section is all about—getting started!

I have included 50 simple plant-based recipes you can make at home, with no special equipment (except a blender or a food processor for a few) and no exotic ingredients. The foods are ones you will recognize, and many of them are comfort foods or "standard" favorites. My goal is to give you options to allow you to continue to eat the foods you love but in a healthier version.

The recipes are all meat, dairy, gluten, and oil-free, except a few recipes that offer options—for example, a few drops of sesame oil to flavor an Asian noodle dish. You can adapt and adjust these recipes to suit your and your family's needs. That is the goal of this entire book—to show you that an anti-inflammatory, intermittent fasting lifestyle is flexible enough to fit into everyone's regimen. And I hope these recipes will prove that it is not only a healthy lifestyle but a tasty one, too!

These recipes are my own, though a few of them have been inspired by great vegan cooks on the many blog sites and channels that I follow. If a recipe is taken from another source, I will list that in the recipe description. I have received permission to use these, and I am grateful for their generosity! That is something that I value about the plant-based community—their willingness and passion for sharing this lifestyle with others in order to bring better health to the planet and its people.

Okay, it's time to get cooking. Bon appétit!

1. BLUEBERRY "GREEN" SMOOTHIE

This is a great way to get in some extra servings of vegetables without being able to taste them. This one is even a hit with the kids!

Servings: 2

Ingredients:

- 2 small frozen bananas
- 2 cups frozen blueberries
- 2 cups unsweetened plant milk
- 2 tbsp almond butter
- 2 handfuls fresh greens (i.e., spinach, kale)
- 2 tbsp ground flax seed or ground chia seeds

Directions:

1. Place all ingredients in the blender, and blend until smooth. May add additional plant milk for desired consistency. Divide between 2 glasses. Drink immediately. Yields 2 servings.

Note: If there will be a delay in drinking, do not add flax or chia seeds until ready to drink, as sitting will thicken the smoothie up dramatically.

2. CHOCOLATE–BANANA SMOOTHIE

When I was growing up, my father had an ice cream shop, and my favorite thing on the menu was the chocolate banana malt. This takes me back to all the joy but not the guilt. It is a delicious, filling, nutritious, naughty-tasting smoothie that you will find yourself coming back to again and again for both breakfast and as a snack.

Servings: 1

Ingredients:

- 1 large ripe banana, frozen
- 1 cup unsweetened plant milk
- 1 ½ tbsp raw cacao powder
- 4 large pitted dates
- 2 tbsp ground flaxseed
- ½–1 cup of ice cubes

Directions:

1. Place all of the ingredients into a blender, and blend until smooth and creamy. Enjoy immediately.

3. EASY AVOCADO TOAST

It's pretty much impossible to go wrong with creamy, delicious avocado toast. This versatile favorite can be a simple breakfast or an elaborate appetizer. Either way, it's sure to be a crowd favorite.

Servings: 2

Ingredients:

- 2 slices whole grain bread, toasted, or 2 pieces of sliced baguette, if serving as an appetizer
- 1 ripe avocado, mashed and divided
- ½ cup red onion, thinly sliced
- 1 tsp sesame seeds or everything bagel seasoning
- 1 tsp lemon juice
- Sea salt and pepper to taste

Toppings: (Optional—the sky's the limit here, really. Whatever sounds good to you will probably be good!)

- thinly ribboned vegetables such as carrots or cucumber pair well with avocado
- chopped cilantro
- pico de gallo
- vegan feta cheese crumbles
- capers
- green onions

- olive oil for drizzling

Directions:

1. Spread ½ of the mashed avocado onto each piece of toast.
2. Layer with onion slices.
3. Add additional optional toppings, as desired.
4. Sprinkle with sesame seeds or Everything bagel seasoning.
5. Squeeze lemon juice over top.
6. Season with salt and pepper to taste.
7. Serve immediately.
8. Enjoy!

4. PEANUT BUTTER OVERNIGHT OATS

Make ahead and put it in the refrigerator for a delicious, satisfying "breakfast on the go." These can be eaten hot or cold, and you can substitute an unlimited variety of add-ins and toppings. This recipe is for one serving, but trust me—you're going to want to make more.

Servings: 1

Ingredients:

- 1/2 cup unsweetened plant milk
- 3/4 tbsp chia seeds
- 2 tbsp natural peanut butter or nut butter of choice
- 1 tbsp maple syrup
- 1/2 cup rolled oats

Toppings (optional):

- sliced banana, strawberries, or raspberries
- flaxseed meal or additional chia seeds
- cacao nibs
- granola

Directions:

1. To a small jar or bowl (with lid), add nut milk, chia seeds, nut butter, and maple syrup. Stir to combine.

2. Add oats and stir again. Press down to make sure oats are fully covered by milk.

3. Cover or seal and put in the refrigerator for at least 6 hours (best overnight!).

4. Remove from refrigerator and enjoy as-is or with toppings of choice (options above).

5. Keeps for up to 3 days in the refrigerator. Do not freeze.

Note: Overnight oats can be heated in a microwave or saucepan. Add more liquid during heating, as needed.

5. BREAKFAST OAT COOKIES

Who says you can't have your cake and eat it too? Or, in this case, cookies. Enjoy these guilt-free for breakfast, or an easy on-the-go snack.

Servings: 9 cookies

Ingredients:

- 1 cup rolled oats
- 1/3 cup almond meal or almond flour
- 3 tbsp dried coconut
- 1 tsp cinnamon
- 1/4 tsp baking soda
- 3 tbsp almond butter
- 3 tbsp maple syrup
- 1 medium ripe banana
- ½ cup slightly mashed fresh berries

Directions:

1. Preheat the oven to 320°F and line a cookie sheet with parchment paper.
2. Place all the ingredients, except berries, in a medium bowl and mix well. Place the mixture in the freezer for 10–15 minutes.

3. Remove from the freezer. Using damp/wet hands, make 9 balls from the mixture and place on cookie sheet.

4. Press down to create cookie shapes. Press a few berries onto the top of each cookie.

5. Bake for 20 minutes until golden brown.

6. Allow them to cool completely before eating.

6. DELICIOUS BANANA OAT PANCAKES

These are healthy, hearty pancakes, but they also work well as a treat or snack. Top with some nut butter to add more protein and healthy fat, and some fresh fruit and you have a well-rounded meal. They store well in the fridge or freezer, and heating them in a dry, hot non-stick pan works best.

Servings: 2

Ingredients:

- 1 cup rolled oats, blended to a fine powder in a blender or food processor
- 1/2 cup plant milk of choice (up to 1 cup for thinner pancakes)
- 1 large banana
- 2 tsp baking powder
- 1 scant tbsp apple cider vinegar
- 1 tsp vanilla extract
- ⅛ tsp salt
- ¼ tsp cinnamon (optional)

Directions:

1. Blend the oats in a blender or food processor until they are a fine powder.
2. Add all the rest of the ingredients and blend until smooth.

3. Allow to sit and thicken for 5–10 minutes.

4. Heat a non-stick pan over medium to medium-high heat.

5. Pour in a scant ¼ cup of batter at a time per pancake.

6. Cook for 2–3 minutes per side. When the pancake begins to bubble on top and releases on its own, flip.

7. Cook on the other side.

8. Repeat, using all the batter.

7. TOFU BREAKFAST SCRAMBLE

This is great for a Sunday brunch or "breakfast for dinner" meal. It is delicious paired with plant-based "sausage," roasted potatoes, peppers, and onions and topped with salsa and vegan sour cream. Kind of a Mexican skillet breakfast meal. Below is the basic scramble recipe.

Servings: 4

Ingredients:

- 1 16 oz block firm or extra-firm tofu
- 2 tbsp nutritional yeast
- 1 tsp garlic powder
- ½ tsp onion powder
- ¼ tsp turmeric
- ¼ tsp dried dill
- 2 tsp soy sauce or tamari
- 2 tbsp unsweetened non-dairy milk
- black salt to taste (optional, but recommended; gives an "egg" flavor)

Directions:

1. Heat a non-stick pan over medium heat.
2. Crumble the tofu by hand directly into the hot pan.

3. Cook for about 5 minutes, stirring occasionally to prevent sticking. Most of the water should evaporate.

4. Add nutritional yeast, garlic powder, onion powder, turmeric, and dill. Stir until well combined and the tofu turns yellow. Cook for 2–3 minutes, stirring frequently.

5. Pour in soy sauce and non-dairy milk, stir well, and cook for about 30 seconds.

6. Serve immediately.

8. SKILLET BREAKFAST HASH

I call this one "refrigerator clean-out hash." You can throw in whatever you have on hand. No need to go out and buy special ingredients. Below are some of my favorites. This goes well with the Tofu Breakfast Scramble—combine for a one-skillet dish.

Servings: 4–6

Ingredients:

- 4 potatoes (Yukon Gold or other non-starchy variety)
- ½ cup yellow bell pepper
- ½ cup green pepper
- ½ cup red bell pepper
- ½ cup orange bell pepper
- ½ cup sweet onion
- 2 cloves garlic, minced
- 2 cups fresh spinach
- ½ cup cremini or Baby Bella mushrooms
- 1 tsp pepper
- ½ tsp salt
- 1 ½ tsp Italian seasoning
- 1 tsp garlic powder

Optional:

- 1-2 tsp of oil for sautéing. If oil-free, omit the oil and use a non-stick skillet
- ½ lb vegan sausage crumbles
- drizzle of maple syrup

Directions:

1. Cut potatoes into small cubes of equal size. Soak in water for 30 minutes.
2. Once the potatoes have soaked for 30 minutes, drain thoroughly and pat dry with a towel.
3. Heat non-stick skillet on medium-high heat. If not oil-free, may use small amount of oil for sautéing.
4. Add the potatoes in a single layer. Depending on the size of the skillet, this may need to be done in batches. DO NOT overcrowd the skillet, or the potatoes will stick.
5. Cook for 2 minutes—do NOT touch during that time!
6. Flip potatoes and cook another 2 minutes.
7. Repeat, and cook for 2 more minutes. Do this until the potatoes have cooked for a total of 10 mins.
8. Reduce heat to medium-low. Add peppers, onion, and garlic. Combine.
9. If adding plant-based sausage, add now.

10. Add salt, pepper, Italian seasoning, and garlic powder. Stir to combine.
11. Add in the spinach and mushrooms and cook for 2 minutes.
12. Add a drizzle of maple syrup and cook until spinach has wilted.
13. Serve immediately.
14. Top with sliced avocado, vegan sour cream, salsa, etc.

9. TOFU BACON

This "bacon" is chewy, salty, smoky, and a great addition to any breakfast, wrap, or sandwich. Can also be cut into small pieces to use as salad or soup topping.

Ingredients:

- 16 oz block extra firm tofu—drained, pressed, and cut into thin slices (⅛ inch thick)

Marinade:

- ½ cup soy sauce or tamari
- 2 tbsp maple syrup
- 2 tbsp tomato paste
- 1 tsp smoked paprika
- 1 tsp liquid smoke
- ¼ tsp black pepper

Directions:

Whisk marinade ingredients together. Place tofu slices in a container, and pour marinade over the slices. Cover and marinate in the refrigerator for a minimum of 1 hour. Overnight is best!

When done marinating:

1. Preheat oven to 375°F.
2. Line baking sheet with parchment paper.
3. Place tofu in single layer on baking sheet. Save marinade.
4. Bake for 20 minutes.
5. Flip and brush with more marinade.
6. Bake an additional 15–20 mins, or until desired crispiness.

10. CHIA SEED PUDDING (OVERNIGHT)

Full of healthy Omega-3 fatty acids, this simple pudding works as a light breakfast or dessert—or anytime you are craving something sweet and creamy. Keep the basic pudding ready in the refrigerator, and fill with optional mix-ins and toppings, depending on your mood!

Servings: 1

Ingredients:

- 1 cup unsweetened plant milk of choice
- 4 tbsp chia seeds
- 1 tbsp maple syrup (optional; may also use another sweetener of choice)
- ½ tsp vanilla

Toppings (optional):

- fresh berries or other fruit
- shaved coconut
- cacao nibs
- granola

Directions:

1. Place the first 4 ingredients into a jar or other container with a tight-fitting lid.

2. Shake or mix until well blended.
3. Leave on the counter for 10–15 minutes, and shake or mix again until ingredients are well combined.
4. Place in the refrigerator overnight.
5. Mix and serve cold, either plain or with optional toppings.

Note: In order to make chocolate chia pudding, you may also add 2 tbsp unsweetened cocoa powder at the time of mixing.

11. "NO TUNA" SALAD SANDWICH

Every now and then, I get a wave of nostalgia and want a tuna sandwich. This recipe hits the spot. If you like everything about a tuna sandwich except the tuna (or the fishy taste), this one's for you. If you actually miss that fish taste, you can add a sheet of toasted nori seaweed to the mix (in the recipe below) to give it a more authentic flavor. This can be used as a sandwich filling, atop greens for a salad, or as a dip/spread for veggies or crackers.

Servings: 2 sandwiches

Ingredients:

Filling:

- 1 15 oz (1 ½ cups) can of chickpeas, rinsed and drained OR 1 cup of unsalted sunflower seeds, roughly chopped
- 1 stalk celery, finely chopped
- ½ cup red onion, finely chopped
- 3 tbsp tahini or vegan mayo
- 1 tbsp maple syrup
- 1 tbsp fresh dill, or 2 tsp dried
- 1 tsp spicy mustard
- 1 tsp fresh parsley, chopped
- ½ sheet nori seaweed, toasted in pan and crumbled into small pieces (Optional, but this will give a "seafood" flavor more closely resembling tuna)

- sea salt and pepper to taste

Sandwich:

- 4 slices whole grain bread, plain or toasted
- 2 large lettuce leaves
- 2 slices tomato
- chopped green onions for garnish

Directions:

1. If using chickpeas, place in a bowl and mash with a large fork or potato masher.
2. Add remaining ingredients through nori. Stir to combine well.
3. Add salt and pepper to taste.
4. Assemble sandwiches.
5. Enjoy!

Note: If using sunflower seeds, either roughly chop them first and then follow the above instructions, or you can place sunflower seeds, celery, and red onion in a food processor and pulse until roughly chopped and combined. Then place all ingredients into a bowl and stir well.

12. VEGAN BLT/A WRAP

This is the classic BLT, elevated to another level with the addition of creamy avocado. This makes a great light lunch, or pairs well with a bowl of soup or chili for a more hearty dinner.

Servings: 2 wraps

Ingredients:

- 2 whole-grain wraps
- ½ of an avocado
- 2 small tomatoes, thinly sliced
- 2 large romaine lettuce leaves
- 6–8 strips Tofu Bacon (see recipe)
- 2 tbsp Creamy Cashew Mayo (see recipe) or vegan mayo of your choice

Directions:

1. Spread whole-grain wraps with vegan mayo.
2. Top with slices of avocado, tomatoes, lettuce, and bacon.
3. Roll up and enjoy!

13. BEAUTIFUL BUDDHA BOWLS

Buddha bowls can be as simple or as complex as you want them to be. They are kind of like salads, but in my opinion, even better. There are no rules, per se—just a tasty combination of ingredients. Choose from each of the categories below, and top with a dressing of your choice.

Ingredients:

Choose your grain:

- brown rice
- quinoa
- millet
- buckwheat
- barley

Choose your veggies:

(Add at least 2 or 3 kinds—but no limit!—of raw, roasted, or steamed veggies)

- carrot
- cucumber
- bell pepper
- mushroom
- tomato
- sweet potato
- avocado

- cauliflower
- pumpkin
- broccoli
- zucchini
- spinach
- kale
- radish
- beets
- bok choy
- snap peas
- corn

Choose your plant-based protein:

- tofu
- tempeh
- beans
- lentils
- edamame
- chickpeas
- falafel (chickpea or fava bean fritter)

Choose your toppings:

- pumpkin seeds
- sesame seeds
- hemp seeds
- kimchi

- sauerkraut
- olives
- sprouts
- pickled ginger
- pickled or fermented vegetables

Choose your dressing:

- tahini dressing
- hummus
- peanut sauce
- ginger, garlic, soy dressing
- any other prepared dressing of choice
- or just a squeeze of lime or some apple cider vinegar

Directions:

1. Combine your choice of the above ingredients in a bowl, mix, and enjoy!

14. FRESH VEGGIE SPRING ROLLS

These are fresh and tasty, and make great appetizers or a light lunch. They are fun to make as a group—provide the wrappers and different fillings, and allow everyone to make their own.

Servings: 2

Ingredients:

- 4 brown rice spring roll wrappers
- variety of vegetables (carrot, cucumber, red onion, bell peppers), cut into thinly sliced sticks
- green onions, chopped
- 4 cilantro sprigs
- 4 mint sprigs
- 4 romaine lettuce leaves
- large plate or pie dish with ½–1 inch of water for dipping spring roll wrappers

Optional:

- 8 basil leaves
- sliced fruit, such as mango or pineapple
- cooked tofu

Directions:

1. Submerge the rice wrapper in water for 10–15 seconds. It will still be firm when removed from the water but will soften up as you assemble the spring roll.
2. Drain off excess water and place the wrapper flat on your counter or cutting board.
3. Place romaine leaf lengthwise onto the 1/3 of the wrapper closest to you. Make sure it does not overhang the sides of the wrapper.
4. Place vegetable slices, tofu if using, green onion pieces, and herbs on top of the lettuce leaf.
5. Fold in the sides of the wrapper, covering the ends of the lettuce leaf and vegetables.
6. Lift the edge of the wrapper closest to you, and pull it up and over the top of the leaf and vegetables.
7. Begin to roll away from you, keeping contents tight, until the spring roll has been completely enclosed, and looks like a small burrito.
8. Repeat with the rest of the wrappers and filling ingredients.
9. Serve with Tasty Thai Peanut Sauce, or Ginger Garlic Sauce for dipping.

15. HEARTY VEGETABLE MINESTRONE SOUP

This soup makes a great lunch or dinner on cold winter days/nights. It is packed with everything you need for a complete one-bowl meal. Pair with some crusty bread and plant-based butter for the ultimate comfort food.

Servings: 8

Ingredients:

- 1 large yellow onion
- 3 cloves of garlic, minced
- 2 large carrots, sliced into rounds
- 3 stalks celery, chopped
- 1 tbsp Italian seasoning
- 1 cup cut fresh or frozen green beans
- 2 cans (3 cups) white beans or red kidney beans
- 1 28-ounce can of plain or fire-roasted tomatoes
- ¼ cup tomato paste
- 4 cups vegetable broth
- 1–2 cups water (to cover ingredients)
- 1 tbsp soy sauce or tamari
- 1 tbsp maple syrup
- 2 tsp garlic powder
- 2 tsp balsamic vinegar
- 1 package whole grain or gluten-free pasta
- 2 cups chopped kale or spinach
- salt and pepper to taste

Directions:

1. In large pot over medium heat, sauté the first five ingredients (onion through Italian seasoning) for 5–6 minutes, until onions are softened.
2. Add green beans and white or red kidney beans and stir well.
3. Add the next eight ingredients (can of tomatoes through balsamic vinegar). Bring to a boil, then reduce heat and simmer for 20–30 mins.
4. Add the pasta, kale or spinach, and salt and pepper, and cook for 10 mins or until pasta is fully cooked.

16. EASY 2-BEAN VEGGIE CHILI

Chili is such a versatile dish. It can stand alone as a stew or soup, or be used as a topping for things like nachos, a baked potato, or a carrot "hot dog." Below is the basic recipe, but feel free to throw in extra vegetables, different types of beans, spicy peppers, plant-based meat alternatives, or whatever your heart desires.

Servings: 4–6

Ingredients:

- 2 cans (15 oz each) black beans, rinsed and drained
- 1 can (15 oz) pinto beans, rinsed and drained
- 2 cups vegetable broth or water
- 1 large can (28 oz) or 2 small cans (15 oz each) diced tomatoes, undrained
- 1 medium red onion, chopped
- 1 large red bell pepper, chopped
- 2 medium carrots, peeled and chopped
- 2 ribs celery, chopped
- ½ teaspoon salt, divided
- 4 cloves garlic, minced
- 2 tbsp chili powder
- 1 tbsp ground cumin
- 1 ½ tsp smoked paprika
- 1 tsp dried oregano

- 1 bay leaf
- 2 tbsp chopped fresh cilantro, plus more for garnishing
- 1–2 teaspoons lime juice, to taste
- optional garnishes: chopped cilantro, diced avocado, crushed tortilla chips, sour cream/yogurt

Directions:

1. Heat soup pot or Dutch oven over medium heat.
2. Add the chopped onion, bell pepper, carrot, celery, and ¼ teaspoon of salt. Add water as needed to keep veggies from sticking. Cook, stirring occasionally until the vegetables are tender and the onion is translucent, about 7 to 10 minutes.
3. Add the garlic, chili powder, cumin, smoked paprika, and oregano. Cook until fragrant while stirring constantly, about 1 minute.
4. Add the beans, vegetable broth, tomatoes, and bay leaf. Stir to combine.
5. Bring to a low boil, then reduce heat to low and simmer for 30 mins.
6. Remove from the heat and remove the bay leaf.
7. Add cilantro, lime, and the rest of the salt to taste.
8. Divide into bowls and top with optional garnishes.

Note: For a thicker consistency, you may add 1 tbsp of cornstarch dissolved in 2 tbsp water (slurry) to the chili and continue to simmer until desired consistency. Alternately, after removing bay leaf, you may blend 1–2 cups of the chili in a blender and then return to the pot.

17. EASY TACO SOUP

This is so simple, inexpensive, and always a crowd-pleaser. It can be a main-dish lunch, or try this soup alongside Mexican Stuffed Bell Peppers for a full, hearty dinner. The flavors are even better the next day after having time to blend.

Ingredients:

- 1 15 oz can of black beans, not drained
- 1 15 oz can of pinto beans, not drained
- 1 15 oz can of kidney beans, not drained
- 1 15 oz can of corn kernels, drained and rinsed
- ½–1 cup sliced black olives
- 1 15 oz can diced tomatoes (with juices) OR large can of Rotel diced tomatoes with green chilies, not drained
- 1 15 oz can tomato sauce
- 1 cup vegetable broth or water
- 1 medium to large onion, diced
- 1 1 oz packet taco seasoning
- 1 1 oz packet dairy-free ranch dressing/seasoning
- 2 tbsp nutritional yeast (optional)

Toppings (optional):

- plant-based sour cream or yogurt
- diced avocado
- crushed tortilla chips

- diced green onion
- chopped fresh cilantro
- jalapeno slices
- plant-based cheddar cheese

Directions:

1. In Dutch oven or large soup pot, sauté onion until softened and starting to brown.
2. Add all the remaining ingredients and bring to a boil.
3. Reduce heat and simmer for 30–45 minutes, stirring occasionally.
4. Serve and garnish with toppings of choice.

18. "CAN'T BELIEVE THERE'S NO DAIRY" POTATO SOUP

The name says it all!

Ingredients:

- 2 lbs of potatoes, peeled and cut into small cubes
- 4 cups vegetable broth
- 1 cup creamy oat milk or full-fat coconut milk
- 1 large onion, diced
- 1 large carrot, diced
- 2 stalks of celery, diced
- 4 cloves of garlic, minced
- 1 bay leaf
- 2 tbsp nutritional yeast (optional)
- 1 tbsp fresh rosemary (or 1 tsp dried)
- 1 tbsp fresh dill (or 1 tsp dried)
- 1 tbsp fresh thyme (or 1 tsp dried)
- 1–2 tsp salt, to taste
- 1 tsp paprika
- ¾ tsp black pepper
- ½ tsp crushed red pepper flakes
- ½ tsp liquid smoke

Garnish:

- Chopped fresh parsley, chives, Tofu Bacon, plant-based sour cream

232 | KARIN FELTMAN, RN

Directions:

1. In a non-stick skillet or Dutch oven over medium heat, sauté onions, carrots, and celery in a bit of vegetable broth until onions become translucent.
2. Add garlic, bay leaf, rosemary, dill, and thyme. Sauté for another 2 minutes or until fragrant.
3. Add potatoes and stir well to combine.
4. Pour in the rest of the vegetable broth, nutritional yeast (if using), salt, pepper, paprika, red pepper flakes, and liquid smoke.
5. Bring to a boil, then reduce heat and simmer until the potatoes are tender, about 20 mins.
6. Remove bay leaf and stir in plant milk.
7. For a thick and creamy soup, place ½ of the soup in a blender. Blend and return to the pot with the rest of the soup.
8. Serve, top with optional garnishes, and enjoy!

19. MEXICAN STUFFED BELL PEPPERS

These peppers are delicious, easy to make, and they freeze and reheat well. They will remind you of the stuffed peppers mom used to make, only better. Feel free to use any kind of bean or vegetable in the filling. This recipe is meant to be a template—but creativity is allowed!

Servings: 4–6

Ingredients:

- 4–5 large bell peppers, any color
- 1 yellow onion, finely chopped
- 4 cloves garlic, minced
- 2 chipotle peppers in adobo sauce, minced
- 1 cup frozen corn
- 1 15 oz can (1 ½ cups) black beans, drained and rinsed
- 1 cup cooked brown rice
- 1 14 oz can diced tomatoes, drained
- ½ cup fresh cilantro, chopped
- salt & pepper to taste

Toppings (optional):

- crushed tortilla chips
- chopped green onion
- vegan sour cream or plain yogurt

- cashew queso
- guacamole
- salsa

Directions:

1. Preheat oven to 350F ֹ
2. Bring 1 gallon of water to a boil in a large pot.
3. Cut off the tops of the bell peppers, about ½ inch from the top. Remove stem and seeds.
4. Place the peppers in the boiling water and cook for 3–4 minutes, until they soften. Remove the peppers from the water, place cut side up, and let cool.
5. Preheat a non-stick skillet over medium heat. Once hot, add the chopped onions and cook until soft and slightly brown, about 5 minutes.
6. Add garlic, chipotle peppers, corn, and black beans. Cook for 2–3 minutes, then transfer the mixture to a large mixing bowl. Add the tomatoes, brown rice, and cilantro to the mixture. Stir well to combine.
7. Arrange the peppers in an 8×8 baking dish and fill with rice mixture. Place in the oven and bake for 35 minutes.
8. Remove from the oven, and top with optional toppings.
9. Serve immediately.

20. HOMESTYLE MAC AND CHEESE

Sometimes, you just need old-school comfort food, and Mac and Cheese is it! Eat as a side dish, or dress it up for a lunch or dinner entree. Add vegetables such as broccoli or serve Southern-style with greens on the side for a nutrition-packed version.

Servings: 4–6

Ingredients:

- 1 package whole grain or gluten-free macaroni pasta
- 1 batch Creamy Queso Sauce (with the addition of tapioca starch or arrowroot powder; see recipe for details)
- Fresh-cracked black pepper

Toppings (optional):

- Tofu Bacon bits (see recipe)
- chopped green onions
- chopped fresh parsley or cilantro
- sauteed mushrooms
- caramelized onions
- vegan sour cream

Directions:

1. Prepare Creamy Queso Sauce. Keep warm.
2. Prepare pasta according to package directions. Drain
3. Gently fold Creamy Queso Sauce into pasta until well coated.
4. Top with optional toppings.
5. Serve immediately.

21. QUICK BROWN RICE NOODLE AND VEGETABLE STIR-FRY

This dish takes just minutes to prepare and makes a good hot main dish or a cold noodle salad. For a bit of spice, serve with Sriracha sauce or Sambal Oelek.

Servings: 2-3

Ingredients:

- 6 oz brown rice noodles, cooked according to package directions
- 1 large carrot, julienned
- 1 zucchini, julienned
- 1/2 cup frozen green peas
- 1 tbsp sesame seeds

Toppings:

- 1 tbsp cilantro, chopped
- 1 tbsp green onion, chopped

Sauce:

- 1 tbsp tahini
- 1 tbsp soy sauce or tamari
- 1 tbsp maple syrup
- 1 tsp white miso paste

- 1 lime, juiced
- few drops of sesame oil, for flavor

Directions:

1. Whisk together sauce ingredients in a small bowl and set aside.
2. Heat a non-stick skillet over medium-high heat until hot. Add carrots and zucchini and cook for 3–4 minutes until beginning to soften, stirring frequently. Add a bit of water or broth as needed to keep from sticking.
3. Add sesame seeds and peas, and cook for another 3–4 minutes.
4. Add noodles and sauce, and cook for 2–3 minutes, until warmed through.
5. Serve immediately, and top with cilantro and green onion.

22. THAI PEANUT VEG STIR-FRY

This dish can be served as a noodle dish, or you can add vegetable broth and eat it as a Ramen-style soup. It is delicious either way.

Servings: 4

Ingredients:

- 1 red bell pepper, thinly sliced
- 1–2 cups purple cabbage, shredded
- 1/2 medium yellow onion, thinly sliced
- 1 1/2 cups shelled edamame (or tofu)
- 2 large handfuls fresh spinach leaves
- 10 oz whole-grain ramen noodles
- 1/2 cup cilantro, chopped
- 2 tbsp roasted peanuts, chopped (optional for topping)

Peanut sauce: (or for ease, may use store-bought Thai peanut sauce)

- 3 tbsp natural peanut butter
- 4 tbsp soy sauce, tamari or coconut aminos
- 3 cloves garlic, crushed
- 3 tsp maple syrup
- 1 lime, juiced
- 1 tsp Sriracha or other hot sauce

Directions:

1. Cook noodles according to package directions.
2. While the noodles are cooking, whisk together peanut sauce ingredients in a small bowl and set aside.
3. Heat a non-stick skillet over medium heat. Sauteé the cabbage, red bell pepper, spinach, onion, and edamame for 2 minutes.
4. Add the peanut sauce to the vegetables and mix well. Cook until the vegetables are fully cooked, approximately 5–7 minutes.
5. Drain the noodles and add to the pan. Stir well to combine.
6. To serve, top with chopped coriander and peanuts, and additional soy sauce or tamari to taste.

23. ITALIAN-STYLE "MEATBALLS"

These "meatballs" are quick, easy, nutritious, delicious, and versatile. You can pair with dipping sauce as an appetizer, pile them on a crusty roll with marinara sauce for a meatball sub, use them to make a better-than-traditional spaghetti with "meatballs," or get creative and make them into a "meatloaf" (notes on that below the recipe). These are tasty hot and cold and have an even better texture and flavor the day after making them.

Ingredients:

- 1 15 oz can white beans, rinsed and drained (or 1½ cups, cooked from dry)
- 1 cup cooked brown rice
- 8 ounces mushrooms, diced small (3 cups)
- 1 medium onion, diced small (2 cups)
- 6 cloves garlic, minced
- ¼ cup sun-dried tomatoes (about 4 to 5 halves), roasted tomatoes or 1 tbsp tomato paste
- 2 tbsp ground flaxseed meal
- 2 tbsp oat flour/ground oats
- 1 tbsp fresh parsley, finely chopped (or parsley flakes)
- 2 tsp Italian seasoning/mixed herbs
- ¾ tsp fennel seed
- 1 tsp garlic powder
- 1 tsp onion powder

- ½ tsp crushed red pepper flakes (or to taste)
- 2 tsp Worcestershire Sauce
- 1 tbsp white wine vinegar
- 1 tsp sea salt and ¼ tsp freshly ground black pepper (or to taste)

Directions:

1. In a small bowl, soak the sun-dried tomatoes in ½ cup hot water for at least 20 minutes to soften. Drain and finely chop.
2. In a nonstick skillet, combine the onion, mushrooms, garlic, fennel, crushed red pepper, parsley, and ¼ cup water; cook on medium heat for 15 minutes, stirring frequently to prevent sticking. (If needed, add water 1 tbsp at a time to prevent sticking.)
3. Add the rest of the ingredients (unless using tomato paste—then add this at the next step). Mix well, season with salt and pepper, and cook an additional 2 to 5 minutes. Remove from heat and let cool for 10 to 15 minutes.
4. Transfer to a large bowl. Add tomato paste at this time, if using. Use a potato masher or your hands to mash the meatball mixture into a cohesive texture.
5. Preheat oven to 350°F; line a baking sheet with parchment paper. Scoop out 2 tablespoons of the mixture, shape it into a ball, and place on the

prepared baking sheet. Repeat until you have 24 meatballs.

6. Bake for 25–35 minutes, until browned on top.

Note: This recipe may also be pressed into a loaf pan and made into a meatloaf instead. Bake covered for 25 mins, then uncover and top with a layer of marinara, ketchup, or BBQ sauce. Return to oven and bake for additional 15 mins.

244 | KARIN FELTMAN, RN

24. EASY-DOES-IT SPAGHETTI (AND "MEATBALLS")

The name says it all. It's easy, and it's spaghetti and "meatballs." What's not to love? This is a dish that is sure to please the whole family.

Ingredients:

Sauce:

- 4 large cloves of garlic, minced
- 2 28 oz cans of peeled, crushed, or diced tomatoes without added salt
- 1 tsp dried or 3 tsp fresh oregano
- 1 bay leaf
- 1 tsp coconut sugar (to cut acidity)
- ¾–1 tsp sea salt (or to taste)
- ½–1 tsp black pepper (or to taste)
- ¼–½ tsp crushed red pepper flakes (or to taste)
- ½ cup fresh basil, chopped (plus 2 tbsp for garnish)
- 2 tbsp nutritional yeast (optional)
- 2 tbsp tomato paste

Note: Alternately, for ease, you may use a jar of prepared pasta sauce of your choice.

Plus:

- 1 package whole grain pasta
- 1 batch of Italian-Style "Meatballs" (see recipe)

Directions:

1. Heat a large pot over medium-low heat. Add 2 tbsp water and garlic. Sauté for 1 minute, stirring constantly, until golden brown.
2. Add tomatoes, oregano, bay leaf, coconut sugar, salt, and crushed red pepper flakes.
3. Bring to a simmer over medium heat. Reduce heat to low and simmer, uncovered, for 30 minutes, stirring occasionally.
4. While the sauce is simmering, cook pasta to package directions. When finished, drain and set aside.
5. Add basil, nutritional yeast, and tomato paste. Reserve 2 tbsp basil for garnish. Cook for an additional 5 minutes.
6. Taste and adjust flavor, adding more salt, pepper, red pepper flakes, etc., as needed.
7. If the sauce is too thick, add water or vegetable stock to thin it.
8. Ladle sauce and Italian Style "Meatballs" over prepared pasta. Top with fresh basil ribbons and vegan parmesan, if desired.

25. DECADENT MUSHROOM STROGANOFF

This dish is rich, creamy, and hearty. It is a perfect meal to serve guests— no one will miss the meat! You can add a bit of vegan "beef-style" bouillon paste or powder if you want a meatier flavor while still being plant-based compliant, but in my opinion, it doesn't need it.

Servings: 4–6

Ingredients:

- 1 lb mixed mushrooms (portobello, cremini, shiitake), stemmed and cut into large pieces
- 1 oz dried porcini mushrooms, soaked in boiling water for 30 mins (save liquid); OR 1 cup veg/mushroom broth
- 2 large shallots or one yellow onion, diced
- 4 cloves garlic, minced
- 2 teaspoons fresh thyme, minced, or 1 tsp dried
- 1 teaspoon fresh rosemary, minced, or ½ tsp dried
- ½ cup dry white wine
- 1 lb whole-grain fettuccine, cooked according to package directions, drained and kept warm
- 1 cup plant-based sour cream
- parsley, chopped, for garnish
- salt and freshly ground black pepper to taste

Directions:

1. Place the shallots/onion in a large skillet and sauté over medium heat for 8 minutes.
2. If not using oil, add water 1 to 2 tbsp at a time to keep from sticking.
3. Add the garlic and thyme, and cook for 1 minute.
4. Stir in mixed mushrooms, salt and pepper, and rosemary. Cook for 10 minutes, stirring occasionally.
5. Add the porcini mushrooms, their soaking liquid (or 1 cup veg/mushroom broth), and the wine. Lower heat to medium-low and cook for 20 minutes.
6. When the stroganoff is finished cooking, stir in sour cream.
7. Add the cooked noodles and toss well.
8. Serve garnished with parsley and fresh-cracked black pepper.

26. VEG-PACKED CHICKPEA "MEATLOAF"

Inspired by Shane Martin

Arguably one of my absolute favorite plant-based cooking blogs is Shane & Simple (shaneandsimple.com). I am thrilled that Shane Martin has given me permission to share this recipe, inspired by his Chickpea Vegan Meatloaf. This version is gluten-free, as I substitute oats for the bread crumbs, but the result is just as yummy. I like this recipe even better the next day, sliced on a sandwich with salt, pepper, and yellow mustard. Enjoy, and please check out Shane's other amazing recipes as well. I have never been disappointed.

Servings: 8 slices

Ingredients:

- 1 large onion, finely chopped
- 2 celery stalks, finely chopped
- 2 medium carrots, finely chopped
- 2 15 oz cans of chickpeas (approx. 3 cups)
- 1 cup rolled oats
- 3 tbsp ground flax seed
- 2 tbsp nutritional yeast (optional; added for nutrition)
- 1 tbsp garlic powder
- ½ tsp ground sage

- ¼ cup soy sauce or tamari
- 2 tbsp vegan Worcestershire sauce
- 2 tbsp ketchup
- 2 tsp liquid smoke
- ½–1 cup BBQ sauce for topping and serving

Directions:

1. Preheat your oven to 375 F :
2. Heat non-stick pan over medium heat. Sauté onions, carrots, and celery until onions are soft. Remove from heat and set aside.
3. Add drained and rinsed chickpeas to a food processor. Pulse a few times. Add remaining ingredients, through liquid smoke. Pulse until well combined. If you do not have food processor, you can mash in large bowl with potato masher, large fork, or your hands.
4. Scoop mixture into a parchment paper-lined or nonstick loaf pan. Firmly and evenly press the mixture into the pan. Cover with aluminum foil and bake for 25 minutes.
5. Take the loaf out of the oven, remove aluminum foil, and spread BBQ sauce on top. Place back in the oven and cook uncovered for an additional 15 minutes.
6. Remove the chickpea meatloaf from the oven and let it cool in the pan for at least 15 minutes before

serving. The longer it sets, the firmer it gets. This is even better on day two!

7. Serve with BBQ sauce.

8. Cover leftovers and store in the fridge for up to 5 days.

27. LUSCIOUS LENTIL SHEPHERD'S PIE

Seriously—this recipe is going to be on your regular rotation. It is simple to make and delicious. It also travels well, so makes a good dish to take to get-togethers. Do not be worried if the lentil mixture seems "soupy" when spooning it into the baking dish. As it bakes, the liquid will absorb into the potatoes and lentils and turn out perfectly in the end.

Servings: 6–8

Ingredients:

Mashed Potatoes:

- 6 large potatoes (about 1 lb)
- ⅓ cup unsweetened plant milk
- ½ teaspoon salt
- Optional: 1 tbsp vegan butter, or olive oil to taste. If not using, add more plant milk as needed for texture

Shepherd's Pie Filling:

- 1 medium onion, finely chopped
- 4 cloves garlic, finely chopped
- 1 large carrot, peeled and finely chopped
- 1 cup mushrooms, chopped
- 1 tbsp dried herbs (thyme, rosemary, mixed herbs, Italian seasoning, or mix of these)
- 1 bay leaf

- 2 ½ cups cooked green or brown lentils (or 1 can)
- 2 tbsp arrowroot powder, or cornstarch
- 3 tbsp soy sauce or tamari
- 1 cup canned crushed tomatoes
- 1 cup vegetable stock
- 1 ½ tsp salt
- 1 tsp black pepper

Directions:

1. Preheat oven to 400°F.
2. Peel the potatoes and cut each into about 6 pieces.
3. Put the chopped potatoes into a large pan and cover with hot water.
4. Add the salt, cover, and bring to a boil. Simmer for about 15 minutes until the potatoes are very tender (check with a fork or knife).
5. Drain and return to the pan. Leave them with the lid off for a few minutes to allow them to steam dry.
6. Add the milk and optional butter/oil to the pan and mash until creamy. Set aside.
7. Heat a nonstick skillet or saucepan over medium heat. Sauté onions, carrot, mushrooms, and garlic, until the onions start to brown.
8. Add the dried herbs, bay leaf, lentils, and arrowroot powder or cornstarch. Stir well.
9. Add the soy sauce and tomatoes, and stir well.

10. Add the vegetable stock and stir again. Bring to a boil, reduce heat, and simmer for 10 mins.

11. Season with salt and pepper, and spoon the lentil mixture into an ovenproof dish.

12. Spoon the mashed potatoes onto the lentil mixture, and spread evenly over the top.

13. If you desire, you may brush with a small amount of melted vegan butter or olive oil for a crispier top.

14. Place ovenproof dish on a baking tray (to protect against dripping inside your oven) and bake for 30 minutes, or until the top is golden and crisp and the lentil mixture is bubbling.

15. Remove from heat and let sit for 15 mins before serving.

28. ZUCCHINI LASAGNA

This lasagna substitutes zucchini for lasagna noodles. It is a fantastic one-pan dish!

Servings: 4

Ingredients:

- 4 medium zucchinis, thinly sliced lengthwise
- 1 24 oz jar pasta sauce of choice
- 1 batch of "Ricotta" Filling (see recipe)
- 1/4 cup vegan mozzarella cheese (Miyokos brand liquid mozzarella works well for this)
- 2 tbsp Vegan Parmesan (see recipe)
- salt and pepper

Directions:

1. Preheat oven to 350°F.
2. Sprinkle each zucchini slice with a little salt and set on a paper towel-lined baking sheet to draw out excess water.
3. Make "ricotta" filling and vegan parmesan, and set aside.
4. Spread ½ cup of pasta sauce on the bottom of the baking dish.
5. Pat zucchini slices dry, and place a layer on top of pasta sauce.

6. Top zucchini slices with 1/3 of the ricotta filling.

7. Top with ¾ cup pasta sauce and sprinkle with vegan parmesan.

8. Repeat with another layer of zucchini, ricotta, sauce, and parmesan.

9. Make a total of 3 full layers.

10. End with a layer of zucchini topped with pasta sauce, vegan mozzarella, and parmesan.

11. Bake for 35–40 minutes, until bubbling and lightly browned on top.

29. "RICOTTA" FILLING

Smooth, creamy, and flavorful- this is one of my favorite "hacks." It is inexpensive, packed with nutrition (especially protein), and hard to distinguish from actual ricotta when it is baked into a dish like lasagna. For sweet dishes calling for ricotta, omit the herbs, garlic, nutritional yeast, and adjust the lemon and salt to taste.

Ingredients:

- 1 block (12–16 oz) extra-firm tofu, drained
- 1 tbsp nutritional yeast
- 3 cloves garlic
- 1/4 cup fresh parsley, chopped
- 4 tbsp vegan parmesan (optional)
- 1 tsp dried Italian seasoning or mixed herbs
- 1 tbsp lemon juice
- ¼ tsp salt, or to taste

Directions:

1. Place all ingredients into a food processor and blend until smooth and creamy.

30. VEGAN PARMESAN

While this doesn't taste exactly like Parmesan, it does have a similar flavor and texture and is delicious sprinkled on Italian dishes, soups, salads, and popcorn.

Ingredients:

- ¾ cup raw unsalted cashews
- 3 tbsp nutritional yeast
- ½ tsp garlic powder
- ¾ tsp salt

Directions:

1. Blend all ingredients together in a bullet or high-speed blender until it becomes a fine powder. Store in the fridge for up to 2 weeks.

31. WHOLE ROASTED CAULIFLOWER

This is a delicious, savory dish that can be a stand-alone main dish and the star of any meal. I love this as the centerpiece of a holiday dinner, but it works equally well as humble weekday fare. It manages to be fancy while still being simple.

Servings: 2-4

Depends on the size of the cauliflower, and whether serving as a main dish or side.

Ingredients:

- 1 medium-sized head of cauliflower

Marinade:

- 2 tbsp olive oil, or vegetable broth to make it oil-free
- 2 tbsp mixed or Italian herbs
- 2 cloves garlic, minced or crushed
- 1 tbsp Worcestershire sauce
- 1 tbsp soy sauce or tamari
- 1 tsp garlic powder
- 1 tsp onion powder
- 1 tsp smoked paprika
- ½ tsp salt
- ½ tsp pepper
- ¼ tsp crushed red pepper flakes

FIT, FIERCE, AND FABULOUS OVER 50! | 259

Directions:

1. Preheat oven to 400°F.
2. Trim off stem and leaves of cauliflower, leaving the head intact.
3. Make some small slits in the cauliflower with a sharp knife.
4. Mix together marinade ingredients in a large ziplock bag, or bowl.
5. If using ziplock bag, place cauliflower into the marinade, seal, and turn and massage until the cauliflower is well coated with marinade. Let sit for up to 1 hour if possible, to ensure the cauliflower is saturated.
6. If using a bowl, put cauliflower into the bowl upside down (core side up) and then pour marinade onto the cauliflower, trying to get it into all of the crevices. Using your hands, coat all surfaces with the marinade until saturated. Let sit for up to 1 hour.
7. Place ½ to 1 inch of water into a shallow baking pan (to help steam and cook the cauliflower while roasting).
8. Place cauliflower, right-side up, into the pan. Reserve leftover marinade. Sprinkle with salt and pepper.
9. Cover with tented foil and place in the oven. Bake for 20 mins.

10. Remove foil, baste with remaining marinade, and place back in the oven to roast for another 25–30 minutes or until tender.

32. CRUNCHY BAKED POTATO WEDGES

These are incredibly addictive. You won't miss the oil. Use these like you would French fries or steak fries. They can be served as a side dish or used as a base layer for a main dish, like potato wedges topped with chili and vegan queso for a fun twist on a loaded baked potato.

Servings: 4-6

Ingredients:

- 4 large baking potatoes
- salt to taste

Optional dipping sauces:

- dijon mustard
- salsa
- sriracha mayo
- tahini dressing
- cashew queso

Directions:

1. Bake or steam whole potatoes until soft but not falling apart.
2. Refrigerate potatoes until cool.
3. Preheat oven to 450°F.

4. Cut cold potatoes into large wedges/fries.
5. Place in a single layer on a parchment paper-lined baking tray and sprinkle with salt.
6. Bake for 20–25 minutes or until brown and crispy on the outside.
7. Enjoy!

Note: May also be made in the air fryer instead of baked in the oven.

33. CREAMED SPINACH

This is nostalgic for me. My mother used to make the most delicious creamed spinach using those rock-hard frozen blocks of chopped spinach from the grocery store. This version has all the taste but a better texture from the fresh spinach. Feel free to use frozen if it works better for you! I like to turn this into a full meal by spooning it over a bed of mashed potatoes. Yum

Servings: 4

Ingredients:

- 2 lbs fresh spinach, chopped (or 2 blocks frozen)
- 1 small onion, diced
- 3 cloves garlic, minced
- ¾ tsp garlic powder
- ½ tsp salt
- ½ tsp black pepper
- ⅛ tsp nutmeg
- 2 tbsp water

Cashew Cream:

- ½ cup soaked cashews
- ½ cup water
- ½ cup plant milk
- ½ tbsp cornstarch or arrowroot powder

- 1 tsp lemon juice
- 1 tsp apple cider vinegar

Directions:

1. Place all ingredients for cashew cream into the blender, and blend until smooth. Set aside.
2. In a non-stick skillet, sauté the onions and garlic for 2 mins, until fragrant.
3. Add spinach, and 2 tbsp of water. Cook until wilted.
4. Pour in cashew cream, and fold into the spinach until well combined and warmed through.
5. Add garlic powder, salt, pepper, and nutmeg.
6. Serve immediately.

34. ROASTED BRUSSELS SPROUTS

Depending on your mood, these make a delicious side dish or even a main dish. I like these dipped in a bit of Sriracha sauce or Dilly Ranch Dip (see recipe). Take them to your next BBQ or tailgate party instead of "wings."

Servings: 6

Ingredients:

- 2 ½ lbs fresh Brussels sprouts, trimmed and cut in half from top to bottom
- 1 ½ tbsp soy sauce, tamari, or coconut aminos
- 1 tbsp maple syrup
- 1 tsp smoked paprika
- 1 tsp cumin
- ½ tsp garlic powder
- salt to taste

Directions:

1. Preheat oven to 400°F.
2. Wash, pat dry, trim, and cut Brussels sprouts into equal halves.
3. Place in a large bowl or ziplock bag (this is best to get them evenly coated with marinade).
4. In a small bowl, mix together the next 5 ingredients (soy sauce through garlic powder). Pour over

Brussels sprouts. Coat completely. If using a ziplock bag, turn in all directions and massage to get the marinade into all the crevices of the sprouts.

5. Once completely coated, lay Brussels sprouts on a parchment paper-lined baking tray in a single layer. Do not pour extra sauce over the top—it will burn.

6. Sprinkle with salt.

7. Bake 15–20 mins, or until tender and just starting to turn dark brown/char.

8. Remove from the oven and enjoy immediately!

35. QUINOA TABBOULEH SALAD

This recipe may be used as a salad, side dish, or main dish. The use of quinoa instead of the traditional bulgur wheat makes this salad gluten-free. Take this along to a BBQ or cookout, and watch it disappear.

Servings: 4

Ingredients:

- 3–4 cups cooked quinoa, any color (yield from 1 cup uncooked)
- 1 cup fresh tomatoes, diced
- 1 cup cucumber, diced
- 1 bell pepper (any color), diced
- 1 medium red onion, diced
- ⅔ cup fresh mint, chopped
- ⅔ cup fresh parsley, chopped
- 2 limes, juiced
- 2 tbsp tahini or 2 tbsp olive oil
- salt and pepper to taste

Directions:

1. Place first 7 ingredients in large bowl.
2. Whisk together lime juice and tahini or oil. Add a bit of water as needed if the tahini is too thick.

3. Pour into the bowl with the rest of the ingredients, and stir well to combine.

4. Season with salt and pepper to taste.

Note: Stores well in the refrigerator for up to 4 days.

36. CREAMY COLESLAW

This one is adjustable to your personal taste. If you like it tangier, add more vinegar. Sweeter? Add more maple syrup. Saltier? You know what to do. This super-simple salad goes well with sandwiches, burgers, BBQ, and cookouts. Nothing says "summer" like coleslaw.

Ingredients:

- 1 large bag (14 oz) of pre-cut coleslaw mix (shredded cabbage, carrots, etc.)
- 1 cup Creamy Cashew Mayo (see recipe)
- 1 tbsp maple syrup
- 2 tbsp apple cider or malt vinegar
- ¼ tsp celery seed
- ½ tsp salt and ¼ tsp pepper (or to taste)

Directions:

1. Put everything into a large mixing bowl, and toss to combine.
2. Chill in the refrigerator for at least one hour before serving.

37. MEXICAN FIESTA PASTA SALAD

Colorful and packed with vegetables, this recipe is great as a light lunch, a side salad, or a take-along potluck dish.

Servings: 4–6

Ingredients:

- 1 16 oz box of whole grain or gluten-free macaroni pasta, cooked according to package directions, drained, rinsed, and cooled
- 1 large red onion, diced
- 1 large celery stalk, diced
- 1 red bell pepper, diced
- 1 yellow or orange bell pepper, diced
- 1 cup Roma tomatoes, diced
- 1 cup frozen corn, thawed
- 1 6 oz can of black olives, sliced (approx. 1 cup)

Dressing:

- 1 cup Creamy Cashew Mayo (see recipe or use vegan mayo of your choice)
- ½ cup mild salsa
- ¼ cup apple cider vinegar
- ⅓ cup maple syrup
- 1 package taco seasoning

Directions:

1. Whisk dressing ingredients together in a small bowl. May add water or more salsa as needed to thin it to desired consistency.
2. Put pasta and vegetables into a large bowl. Top with dressing and mix well to combine.
3. Place in fridge for a minimum of 2 hours—but flavors will blend better if left overnight.

Note: Gluten-free noodles are usually best eaten the same day, as they sometimes develop a "tough" texture when left until the next day. This can vary from pasta to pasta.

38. 3-BEAN SALAD

This classic salad has always been plant-based, so it tastes just like you remember! It is packed with protein and can be used as a side dish or as a main salad.

Servings: 6

Ingredients:

- 1 15 oz can chickpeas (garbanzo beans), drained and rinsed
- 1 15 oz can dark red kidney beans, drained and rinsed
- 2 cups fresh green beans, cut into 1-inch pieces
- 1 cup (or 2 stalks) celery, finely diced
- ½–1 cup (to taste) red onion, finely diced
- 4 tbsp fresh parsley, coarsely chopped
- 6 tbsp apple cider vinegar
- 1 tbsp tahini (or olive oil, if not oil-free)
- 1 tbsp maple syrup
- ½ tsp salt
- ¼ tsp black pepper

Directions:

1. In a small pot of boiling water, cook green beans for 2 minutes.

2. Remove green beans from the water and place them in a bowl of ice water to stop cooking.

3. Place all the beans, celery, onion, and parsley in a mixing bowl. Stir to combine.

4. In a small bowl, whisk together apple cider vinegar, tahini (or oil), maple syrup, salt, and pepper. Pour over the bean mixture and toss to combine.

5. Cover and place in refrigerator for a minimum of 2 hours.

Note: Keeps in the fridge for several days.

274 | KARIN FELTMAN, RN

39. CLASSIC POTATO SALAD

We all have our potato salad preferences. I like mine salty, tart, and mustardy. Some like it sweet. Use this basic recipe, and tweak it how you like it by adding or omitting ingredients to your taste. I also like to dust mine with a bit of Kala Namak (black salt) for an eggy flavor since my mom always put egg slices on top of hers.

Ingredients:

- 2 ½–3 lbs of potatoes, peeled and cut into small cubes
- 4 green onions, white and green parts, diced
- 2 stalks celery, diced
- 1–1 ½ cups cashew or tofu mayo (see recipe) or vegan mayo of choice
- 2 tsp apple cider vinegar or juice of ½ a lemon
- 1 tsp yellow mustard
- ½ tsp celery seed
- ½ tsp salt or to taste
- ½ tsp black pepper
- ¼ cup dill or sweet relish (optional)
- paprika or fresh dill (optional)

Directions:

1. Boil potatoes for 15–20 minutes or until fork-tender.
2. Remove from heat, drain, and cool.
3. In a small bowl, mix mayo, relish (if using), vinegar, yellow mustard, celery seed, salt, and pepper. If too thick, add water or lemon juice 1 tbsp at a time until desired thickness is reached. If too thin, add more mayo.
4. Place potatoes, celery, and onion into a large bowl. Top with mayo mixture. Toss to combine.
5. Adjust salt and pepper to taste.
6. Dust with paprika or sprinkle with fresh dill (optional).
7. Cover and place in the refrigerator for a minimum of 2 hours.

40. BROCCOLI RAISIN SALAD

This is one of my all-time favorite salads since going plant-based. It is crunchy, sweet, salty, smoky, and creamy all at once. It satisfies me on so many levels. Enjoy!

Servings: 6–8

Ingredients:

- 6–8 cups broccoli, cut into small florets
- 1 cup red onion, diced
- ¾ cup raisins or dried cranberries
- ½ cup slivered almonds, lightly pan-toasted
- ⅓ cup tofu bacon, cut into small pieces (optional but delicious)

Dressing:

- 1 ½ cups cashew or tofu mayo (or vegan mayo of your choice)
- 2 tbsp apple cider vinegar
- 2 tbsp maple syrup
- ½ tsp salt
- ½ tsp liquid smoke
- ¼ tsp black pepper

Directions:

1. Whisk together all dressing ingredients in a small bowl. Set aside.
2. Place broccoli in a pan of boiling water for 1 minute. Remove and immediately place in a bowl of ice water to stop cooking. (This will give your broccoli a great texture and a lovely bright green color).
3. Drain broccoli and place in a large mixing bowl.
4. Add onion, raisins or cranberries, almonds, and tofu bacon if using.
5. Top with dressing and toss well to combine.
6. Cover and put in the refrigerator for at least 1 hour. Best if served chilled.

41. BROWN RICE KHIR (RICE PUDDING)

This is a slightly sweet, creamy, healthy version of a South Asian favorite. It can be eaten as a breakfast pudding or dessert. It is made with brown rice instead of traditional white rice. Drizzle with maple syrup or a dollop of date paste when serving if more sweetness is desired.

Servings: 4–6

Ingredients:

- 3 cups cooked brown rice
- 2 cups unsweetened plant milk
- 1 cinnamon stick
- 2 green cardamom pods (or ⅛ tsp ground cardamom)
- 1 star anise
- ⅛ to ¼ teaspoon ground cloves, to taste
- 1 cup dates, pitted and chopped
- 1 tart apple (such as Granny Smith), cored and chopped
- ¼ cup raisins
- salt to taste
- ¼ cup slivered, toasted almonds

Directions:

1. Combine the rice, almond milk, cinnamon stick, cloves, cardamom, star anise, and dates in a medium saucepan and cook, stirring occasionally, over medium-low heat for 12 minutes or until the mixture thickens.
2. Remove the cinnamon stick, cardamom pods, and star anise. Add the apple, raisins, and salt. Stir to combine.
3. Serve garnished with toasted almonds.

42. GUILT-FREE APPLE CRISP

This is definitely a comfort-food dessert. The topping is slightly less crunchy than the oil-laden versions, but it is no less satisfying. This is perfect on cold winter nights. For an occasional extra treat, try topping it with plant-based ice cream. À la mode!

Servings: 6

Ingredients:

Filling:

- 6 apples, cut into thin slices or small chunks (Common varieties for apple crisp include Granny Smith, Golden Delicious, and Honey Crisp, though any apple will work)
- ½ cup water
- 3 tbsp maple syrup
- 1 tbsp lemon juice
- 2 tsp cinnamon (or 1 tsp cinnamon and 1 tsp allspice)
- ½ tsp salt
- ¼ tsp nutmeg
- 2 tbsp arrowroot powder or cornstarch

Crisp Topping:

- 1 cup gluten-free flour
- 1 cup rolled oats

- ½ cup maple syrup
- 1 tsp cinnamon
- ½ tsp baking powder
- ½ tsp salt

Directions:

1. Preheat oven to 350°F.
2. Place dry topping ingredients in a bowl and stir well to combine.
3. Add the maple syrup and stir to combine. If large clumps form, break up into smaller chunks. Set aside.
4. In non-stick skillet over medium-low heat, cook all of the filling ingredients except arrowroot powder/cornstarch until apples are softened, 5–7 minutes.
5. Add water as needed to prevent sticking.
6. Add arrowroot powder or cornstarch and cook another 2–3 minutes, until thickened.
7. If needed, add more water so that there is a "sauce" with the apples.
8. Pour into baking dish and top with crisp topping mixture. Use fingers to break up the topping and spread evenly over apples.
9. Bake, uncovered, for 30–35 minutes, or until bubbly and top is golden brown.
10. Let cool for 5–10 mins before serving.

43. STRAWBERRY CHIA SEED JAM

This makes an excellent replacement for traditional, sugar-laden jams and jellies. You can use another berry instead of strawberries or try mixing them for a unique mixed-berry jam. I love this on top of the Delicious Banana Oat Pancakes. If you find that it is too concentrated or you would like to make it into more of a syrup than a thick jam, you can add some water or fruit juice to the final product at any time before putting it into the fridge. I have even done it the next day with good results.

Ingredients:

- 2 cups fresh or frozen strawberries, roughly chopped
- 2 tbsp chia seeds
- 1 tbsp lemon juice or apple juice
- 2 tbsp maple syrup (optional for added sweetness)
- ½ tsp vanilla

Directions:

1. Heat fruit, maple syrup, and lemon or apple juice in a saucepan on medium heat for 5–7 minutes, stirring frequently until the fruit begins to break down.
2. Use a large fork or potato masher to mash the fruit into desired jam texture.
3. Remove from heat.

4. Stir in chia seeds and vanilla.

5. Let cool at room temperature, stirring at 15 minutes and again at 30 minutes.

6. Store in a tightly sealed jar or container in the fridge for 5–7 days.

44. SUNDRIED TOMATO HUMMUS

Who doesn't love hummus? It is a great snack and adds both protein and healthy fats to your diet. Try this delicious version, or add other add-ins of your choice in place of the sundried tomatoes. Olives, capers, or roasted garlic work well. Serve with fresh vegetables or whole-grain crackers for dipping. Also delicious as an addition to sandwiches, wraps, or as a salad dressing.

Servings: 8

Ingredients:

- 1 15 oz can chickpeas (1 ½ cups), drained and rinsed
- ¼ cup sundried tomatoes, soaked for 30 mins in hot water
- 2 cloves garlic
- ½ a lemon, juiced
- 2 tbsp tahini
- ½ tsp salt
- ¼ cup water (as needed for texture)
- more chopped sundried tomatoes or parsley for serving (optional)

Directions:

1. Place all ingredients except water into a food processor or high-speed blender.
2. Blend until creamy. Stop once or twice to scrape down the sides.
3. If the texture is too thick, add water a little at a time until desired consistency is reached.
4. Store in the refrigerator for up to 5 days.

45. CREAMY QUESO SAUCE

This sauce is delicious over cooked vegetables, as a dip, over pasta to make a vegan "mac and cheese," and more. Use anywhere you would use cheese sauce. To make it into queso, stir in salsa after heating.

Servings: 4

Ingredients:

- 1 cup potato, peeled and cut into large chunks
- ¾ cup carrot, peeled and cut into chunks
- heaping ½ cup of raw cashews (if nut-free, can substitute ½ cup of rolled oats)
- 2 large cloves garlic
- ½ cup onion, roughly chopped
- 1 tsp salt
- ¼ tsp black pepper
- 4 cups water
- ¼ tsp turmeric
- 1 tsp Dijon mustard
- 1 tsp smoked paprika
- 2 tbsp nutritional yeast
- 1 tbsp arrowroot powder or tapioca starch (optional)

Directions:

1. Place the first 8 ingredients (through water) into a large pan with a lid, and bring to a boil. Reduce heat and simmer until potatoes and carrots are completely soft.
2. Remove from heat and allow to cool for 10 minutes.
3. Drain the mixture but keep the cooking water.
4. Place the veggie mix into a blender, and slowly add reserved cooking water until it reaches the desired consistency.
5. Add turmeric, Dijon mustard, paprika, and nutritional yeast and blend until smooth and creamy.
6. If you would like the sauce to have a thicker, "stretchier" texture, add arrowroot powder or tapioca starch at this time. Blend again until well combined. Then add to a pan and reheat. It will thicken as it heats.

46. CREAMY CASHEW MAYO

This makes an excellent base for dressings, sauces, and spreads. Use it just like you would regular mayo. You can use tofu if you prefer a nut-free version. Keep in mind that cashews are high in calories, so use sparingly if you are trying to lose weight.

Servings: 8

Ingredients:

- 1 cup cashews, soaked overnight in water, or boiled for 30 mins then drained
- ½ cup water
- 2 tbsp lemon juice
- 1 tsp Dijon mustard
- 1 tsp onion powder
- 1 tsp garlic powder
- ¼ tsp salt
- 1 tsp nutritional yeast (optional)

Directions:

1. Blend all ingredients in a high-speed blender until smooth and creamy. Taste and adjust with more salt or lemon juice as needed.
2. Keep in a jar or container with a lid in the refrigerator. Will keep for several days, if not longer.

Note: May substitute tofu for cashews for a nut-free version, but start out by blending without water and add as needed for texture.

47. EASY-PEASY TAHINI DRESSING

Use as a dressing on salads, Buddha Bowls, as a dip with Falafel, and more.

Servings: 5-6

Ingredients:

- ⅓ cup tahini
- 1 medium lemon, juiced (approx. 3 Tbsp)
- 1 tbsp maple syrup
- 1 tsp onion powder
- 1 tsp garlic powder
- ½ tsp salt
- 6–8 tbsp cold water

Directions:

1. Place first 6 ingredients (through salt) in small bowl.
2. Whisk to combine. Add water, a little at a time, until you reach the desired consistency. The colder the water, the creamier your dressing will be.

48. DILLY RANCH DIP/DRESSING

This can be used in the same way you would use regular ranch dip or dressing. A thicker consistency works best for dips, and thinner may be used as a dressing on salads or Buddha bowls.

Servings: 4-6

Ingredients:

- 1 package silken tofu
- 2 cloves fresh garlic
- 2 tbsp fresh lemon juice
- 1 tbsp apple cider vinegar
- 1 tbsp dried dill (or ¼ cup fresh)
- 1 tbsp dried parsley (or ¼ cup fresh)
- 2 tsp garlic powder
- 2 tsp onion powder
- 1 tsp dried oregano (or 1 tbsp fresh)
- ½–1 tsp salt (to taste)
- ½ tsp black pepper
- unsweetened plant milk (up to 1 cup) for desired consistency
- 1 tbsp nutritional yeast (optional)

Directions:

1. Place all ingredients except milk in a blender. Blend until well combined.
2. Add plant milk gradually, as needed to achieve desired consistency.

49. GINGER GARLIC SAUCE

I love this sauce on just about everything! It is delicious on noodles, fried rice, buddha bowls, in soup, or as a dip for spring rolls or other finger foods. For a spicy version, add some crushed chili flakes, hot peppers or your favorite hot sauce.

Ingredients:

- ½ cup soy sauce or tamari
- 2 tbsp rice vinegar
- 2 tbsp fresh lemon juice
- 2 cloves garlic
- 2 tbsp minced or grated ginger
- 2 tbsp chopped green onion
- 2 tbsp chopped cilantro
- 1–2 tsp coconut sugar (optional)
- 1–2 tsp sesame oil (optional; omit if oil-free)

Directions:

1. Place first 7 ingredients (through oil) in blender, or whisk vigorously by hand until well combined.
2. Add green onion and cilantro. Mix well and serve.

50. TASTY THAI PEANUT SAUCE

This sauce is good with spring rolls, stir-fries, and on Buddha bowls. It can be turned into a dipping sauce or dressing, depending on your needs. Just adjust the consistency using water or soy sauce/tamari.

Ingredients:

- ½ cup natural peanut butter (or almond butter)
- 2 tbsp soy sauce or tamari
- 2 tbsp maple syrup
- 2 tbsp fresh-squeezed lime juice
- 1 tbsp rice vinegar
- 1 tbsp grated ginger
- 3 cloves garlic, minced or crushed into a paste
- 1 tsp Sriracha or Sambal Oelek (or other chili sauce of choice), or to taste
- water to desired consistency

Directions:

1. Whisk all ingredients in a medium-sized bowl to combine.
2. Add water a little at a time until desired consistency is reached. Make it thicker for use as a dip and thinner as a dressing.

REFERENCES

Abelsson, A. (2022, March 3). *Intermittent fasting: When to work out.* StrengthLog. https://www.strengthlog.com/intermittent-fasting-when-to-work-out/

Alexander, H. (2019, November). *5 benefits of a plant-based diet.* MD Anderson Cancer Center. https://www.mdanderson.org/publications/focused-on-health/5-benefits-of-a-plant-based-diet.h20-1592991.html

Alhamdan, B. A., Garcia-Alvarez, A., Alzahrnai, A. H., Karanxha, J., Stretchberry, D. R., Contrera, K. J., Utria, A. F., & Cheskin, L. J. (2016). Alternate-day versus daily energy restriction diets: Which is more effective for weight loss? A systematic review and meta-analysis. *Obesity Science & Practice, 2*(3), 293–302. https://doi.org/10.1002/osp4.52

Allison, L. (2022, February 24). How to live longer: The different effects of fasting on men and women. *Longevity.Technology Lifestyle | Health, Fitness & Technology.* https://longevity.technology/lifestyle/how-to-live-longer-the-different-effects-of-fasting-on-men-and-women/

Alrowaili, M. G., Hussein, A. M., Eid, E. A., Serria, M. S., Abdellatif, H., & Sakr, H. F. (2021). Effect of intermittent fasting on glucose homeostasis and bone remodeling in glucocorticoid-induced osteoporosis rat model. *Journal of Bone Metabolism, 28*(4), 307–316. https://doi.org/10.11005/jbm.2021.28.4.307

Anderson, M. (2020, February). *What is disordered eating?* Eatright. https://www.eatright.org/health/diseases-and-conditions/eating-disorders/what-is-disordered-eating

Ansley Hill, RD, LD. (2019, July 8). *How to meal plan: 23 helpful tips.* Healthline; Healthline Media. https://www.healthline.com/nutrition/meal-prep-tips

Anti-inflammatory diet – made easy. (2020, September 1). Arthritis NSW. https://www.arthritisnsw.org.au/anti-inflammatory-diet-made-easy/

Ballard, J. (2020, February 24). *Americans say this popular diet is effective and inexpensive.* YouGov. https://today.yougov.com/topics/consumer/articles-reports/2020/02/24/most-effective-diet-intermittent-fasting-poll

Bandurski, K. (2021, June 1). *The ultimate plant-based grocery list*. Taste of Home. https://www.tasteofhome.com/article/plant-based-diet-grocery-list/

Basaraba, S. (2022, January 18). *What Is Intermittent fasting?* Verywell Fit. https://www.verywellfit.com/overview-intermittent-fasting-2223396

Bascom, E. (2022, August 23). *Time-restricted eating starting early in the morning offers benefits*. Healio. https://www.healio.com/news/primary-care/20220823/timerestricted-eating-starting-early-in-the-morning-offers-benefits

Bedosky, L. (2022, March 28). *Meal planning 101: A complete beginner's guide to meal prep*. EverydayHealth. https://www.everydayhealth.com/diet-nutrition/meal-planning/

Bellisle, F., McDevitt, R., & Prentice, A. M. (1997). Meal frequency and energy balance. *The British Journal of Nutrition, 77 Suppl 1*, S57-70. https://doi.org/10.1079/bjn19970104

Beth - Budget Bytes. (n.d.). *Meal prep 101: A beginners guide to meal prepping*. Budget Bytes. https://www.budgetbytes.com/meal-prep-101-a-beginners-guide/

Bjarnadottir, A. (2018a). *The beginner's guide to the 5:2 diet*. Healthline. https://www.healthline.com/nutrition/the-5-2-diet-guide

Bjarnadottir, A. (2018b, October 3). *The 5 best calorie counter websites and apps*. Healthline. https://www.healthline.com/nutrition/5-best-calorie-counters

Bjarnadottir, A., & Kubala, J. (2020, August 4). *Alternate-Day fasting*. Healthline. https://www.healthline.com/nutrition/alternate-day-fasting-guide

Boulware, T. (2021, July 27). *History of fasting*. Deer Lake Lodge Spa Resort. https://deerlakelodge.com/blog/history-of-fasting

Brewer, A. (2022, November). *Intermittent fasting male vs female*. FastingApps. https://fastingapps.com/intermittent-fasting-male-vs-female/

Browning, J. D., Baxter, J., Satapati, S., & Burgess, S. C. (2011). The effect of short-term fasting on liver and skeletal muscle lipid, glucose, and energy metabolism in healthy women and men. *Journal of Lipid Research, 53*(3), 577–586. https://doi.org/10.1194/jlr.p020867

Butler, N. (2020, January 20). *One meal a day: Health benefits and risks.* MedicalNewsToday. https://www.medicalnewstoday.com/articles/320125

Byakodi, R. (2021a, September 6). *Vegan intermittent fasting: 10 tips on how to do it right.* 21 Day Hero. https://21dayhero.com/vegan-intermittent-fasting/

Byakodi, R. (2021b, December 17). *Dirty fast vs clean fast: A beginners guide.* 21 Day Hero. https://21dayhero.com/dirty-fast-vs-clean-fast/

Byakodi, R. (2022, October 19). *What to eat during intermittent fasting: A full guide.* 21 Day Hero. https://21dayhero.com/intermittent-fasting-what-to-eat/

Caldwell, N. (n.d.). *10 benefits of a plant-based diet.* Thistle. https://www.thistle.co/learn/thistle-thoughts/10-benefits-of-a-plant-based-diet

Capó, E. (2021, October 25). *Plant-Based grocery shopping guide.* Center for Nutrition Studies. https://nutritionstudies.org/plant-based-grocery-shopping-guide/

Capritto, A. (2019, February 18). *Should you try the warrior diet?* Verywell Fit. https://www.verywellfit.com/the-warrior-diet-4684768

Capritto, A. (2021, April 23). *Find out why some are fasting to slim down.* Verywell Fit. https://www.verywellfit.com/5-2-diet-pros-cons-and-how-it-works-4770014

Castaneda, R. (2022, October 19). *Intermittent fasting: Foods to eat and avoid.* US News & World Report; U.S. News & World Report. https://health.usnews.com/wellness/food/articles/intermittent-fasting-foods-to-eat-and-avoid

Center for Food Safety and Applied Nutrition. (2020, November 3). *Food allergies.* FDA. https://www.fda.gov/food/food-labeling-nutrition/food-allergies

Chan, T. (2020, October 6). *Clean vs. dirty intermittent fasting.* Simple.life Blog. https://simple.life/blog/dirty-fasting/

Cho, D. J. (2020, January 22). *Stars who've found success with intermittent fasting.* People. https://people.com/health/stars-who-do-intermittent-fasting/

Clem, J., & Barthel, B. (2021). A look at plant-based diets. *Missouri Medicine, 118*(3), 233–238. https://www.ncbi.nlm.nih.gov/pmc/articles/PMC8210981/

Cleveland Clinic. (n.d.). *Autophagy: Definition, process, fasting & signs.* Cleveland Clinic. https://my.clevelandclinic.org/health/articles/24058-autophagy

Clinical Dietetics Team. (2017, May). *Myths and facts about intermittent fasting.* Cleveland Clinic Abu Dhabi. https://www.clevelandclinicabudhabi.ae/en/health-byte/pages/myths-and-facts-about-intermittent-fasting.aspx

Corey, A. (2022, April 30). *Vegan intermittent fasting (A beginner's guide).* Keeping the Peas. https://www.keepingthepeas.com/vegan-intermittent-fasting/

Crawford, E. (2020, June 16). *IFIC: Intermittent fasting replaces clean eating as most popular diet, presents marketing challenges.* FoodNavigator-USA. https://www.foodnavigator-usa.com/Article/2020/06/16/IFIC-Intermittent-fasting-replaces-clean-eating-as-most-popular-diet-presents-marketing-challenges

Danielle. (2022, April 21). *The importance of meal planning: 3 reasons to meal plan weekly.* Project Meal Plan. https://projectmealplan.com/importance-of-meal-planning/

Disordered eating. (n.d.). Butterfly Foundation. https://butterfly.org.au/eating-disorders/eating-disorders-explained/disordered-eating/

Disordered eating. (2019). Kelty Eating Disorders. https://keltyeatingdisorders.ca/types-of-disorders/disordered-eating/

Disordered eating or eating disorder: What's the difference? (2014, February 23). Psychology Today. https://www.psychologytoday.com/us/blog/contemporary-psychoanalysis-in-action/201402/disordered-eating-or-eating-disorder-what-s-the

Disordered eating vs. eating disorders: What's the tipping point? (2019, August 28). The Emily Program. https://www.emilyprogram.com/blog/disordered-eating-vs-eating-disorders-whats-the-tipping-point/

Dogra, T. (2022, January 27). *5 myths busted around intermittent fasting.* Slurrp. https://www.slurrp.com/article/intermittent-fasting-myths-busted-1641913159096

Dolgoff, S. (2021, February 26). *The majority of women in America have disordered eating — many without even knowing it.* Good Housekeeping. https://www.goodhousekeeping.com/health/diet-nutrition/a35036505/what-is-disordered-eating/

Downing, D. (2022, November 3). *How women's bodies change with age: 30, 40, 50 & beyond.* Canyon Ranch. https://www.canyonranch.com/well-stated/post/a-womans-changing-body/

Eckelkamp, S. (2022, May 31). *Your definitive guide to intermittent fasting.* MindBodyGreen. https://www.mindbodygreen.com/articles/your-definitive-guide-to-intermittent-fasting

Editorial Team. (2021, December 21). *Can I exercise while intermittent fasting?* TheHealthSite. https://www.thehealthsite.com/fitness/exercising-while-intermittent-fasting-dos-and-donts-853296/

Edwards, T. (2021, June 16). *Beginners guide to plant-based grocery shopping.* EatPlant-Based. https://eatplant-based.com/beginners-guide-to-plant-based-grocery-shopping/

86 inspirational quotes for 50-year-old women. (2020, June 19). Aging Greatly. https://aginggreatly.com/inspirational-quotes-for-50-year-old-women/

Elflein, J. (2022, February 18). *Topic: Obesity worldwide.* Statista. https://www.statista.com/topics/9037/obesity-worldwide/

Ellis, S. (2022, June 16). *How should you exercise while you're intermittent fasting? Doctors weigh in.* MindBodyGreen. https://www.mindbodygreen.com/articles/how-to-exercise-while-intermittent-fasting

Encyclopaedia Britannica 2022/11/12. (2019). Fasting. In *Encyclopædia Britannica.* https://www.britannica.com/topic/fasting

Endicott, L. (2020, January 14). *Is intermittent fasting healthy for women?* Simple.life Blog. https://simple.life/blog/intermittent-fasting-for-womens-health/

English, N. (2019, June 7). *Does intermittent fasting affect women differently than men?* BarBend. https://barbend.com/intermittent-fasting-women/

Etudo, M. (2021, April 26). *What is disordered eating?* Verywell Health. https://www.verywellhealth.com/disordered-eating-5095720

Fantozzi, J. (2020, March 13). *30 food facts that will blow your mind.* Insider. https://www.insider.com/amazing-food-facts-2017-12

Faris, M. A.-I. E., Kacimi, S., Al-Kurd, R. A., Fararjeh, M. A., Bustanji, Y. K., Mohammad, M. K., & Salem, M. L. (2012). Intermittent fasting during Ramadan attenuates proinflammatory cytokines and immune cells in healthy subjects. *Nutrition Research, 32*(12), 947–955. https://doi.org/10.1016/j.nutres.2012.06.021

Fasting. (n.d.). New World Encyclopedia. https://www.newworldencyclopedia.org/entry/Fasting

Feng, J., Zhang, S., Li, W., Bai, T., Liu, Y., & Chang, X. (2022). Intermittent fasting to the eye: A new dimension involved in physiological and pathological changes. *Frontiers in Medicine, 9*. https://doi.org/10.3389/fmed. 2022.867624

FitPro Team. (2020, October 23). *Intermittent fasting men vs. women*. FitPro Blog. https://www.fitpro.com/blog/intermittent-fasting-men-vs-women/

5 bestthings. (2021, September 2). *How to intermittent fast & have a social life*. 5 Best Things. https://5bestthings.com/how-to-intermittent-fast-have-a-social-life/

5 questions about intermittent fasting. (n.d.). NIH MedlinePlus Magazine. https://magazine.medlineplus.gov/article/5-questions-about-intermittent-fasting

Fletcher, J. (2020, January 3). *Anti-inflammatory diet: Food list and tips*. Medical News Today. https://www.medicalnewstoday.com/articles/320233

4 supplements you must have when you do intermittent fasting. (2020, June 18). The Times of India. https://timesofindia.indiatimes.com/lifestyle/health-fitness/diet/4-supplements-you-must-have-when-you-do-intermittent-fasting/photostory/76425872.cms?picid=76426108

Frey, M. (2020, September 30). *Pros and cons of intermittent fasting*. Verywell Fit. https://www.verywellfit.com/intermittent-fasting-pros-and-cons-4688805

Frysh, P. (2021, May 7). *Caloric deficit: What to know*. WebMD. https://www.webmd.com/diet/calorie-deficit

Fuentes, L. (2022, August 12). *Are you eating enough while intermittent fasting?* Laura Fuentes. https://www.laurafuentes.com/calories-intermittent-fasting/

Fuller, K. (2022, June 28). *Difference between disordered eating and eating disorders*. Verywell Mind. https://www.verywellmind.com/difference-between-disordered-eating-and-eating-disorders-5184548

Gál, K. (2022, January 3). *The best intermittent fasting strategies for women*. Dr. Robert Kiltz. https://www.doctorkiltz.com/intermittent-fasting-for-women/

Gather, H. (2021, October 19). *Do vitamins break a fast? The best supplements for fasting*. Hunter and Gather Foods. https://hunterandgatherfoods.com/blogs/real-food-lifestyle/do-vitamins-break-a-fast

Goodson, A. (2022, May 20). *Soy protein: Good or bad?* Healthline; Healthline Media. https://www.healthline.com/nutrition/soy-protein-good-or-bad

Gordon, B. (2022, August). *3 strategies for successful meal planning.* Eatright. https://www.eatright.org/food/planning-and-prep/smart-shopping/3-strategies-for-successful-meal-planning

*Gottberg, K. (2017, April 27). 50 of the best positive aging quotes I could find. SMART Living 365. https://www.smartliving365.com/50-best-positive-aging-quotes-find/*Groth, L. (2021, March 9). *25 ways your body changes after 50.* Yahoo. https://www.yahoo.com/lifestyle/25-ways-body-changes-50-141510280.html

Gudden, J., Arias Vasquez, A., & Bloemendaal, M. (2021). The effects of intermittent fasting on brain and cognitive function. *Nutrients, 13*(9), 3166. https://doi.org/10.3390/nu13093166

Gunnars, K. (2019, July 22). *11 myths about fasting and meal frequency.* Healthline; Healthline Media. https://www.healthline.com/nutrition/11-myths-fasting-and-meal-frequency

Gunnars, K. (2020a, January 1). *6 popular ways to do intermittent fasting.* Healthline. https://www.healthline.com/nutrition/6-ways-to-do-intermittent-fasting

Gunnars, K. (2020b, April 20). *Intermittent fasting 101 — the ultimate beginner's guide.* Healthline. https://www.healthline.com/nutrition/intermittent-fasting-guide

Harvard School of Public Health. (2018, January 19). *Diet review: Intermittent fasting for weight loss.* The Nutrition Source. https://www.hsph.harvard.edu/nutritionsource/healthy-weight/diet-reviews/intermittent-fasting/

Heilbronn, L. K., Civitarese, A. E., Bogacka, I., Smith, S. R., Hulver, M., & Ravussin, E. (2005). Glucose tolerance and skeletal muscle gene expression in response to alternate day fasting. *Obesity Research, 13*(3), 574–581. https://doi.org/10.1038/oby.2005.61

Heilbronn, L. K., Smith, S. R., Martin, C. K., Anton, S. D., & Ravussin, E. (2005). Alternate-day fasting in nonobese subjects: Effects on body weight, body composition, and energy metabolism. *The American Journal of Clinical Nutrition, 81*(1), 69–73. https://doi.org/10.1093/ajcn/81.1.69

Henry Ford Health Staff. (2020, July 13). *The health benefits of an anti-inflammatory diet.* Henry Ford. https://www.henryford.com/blog/2020/07/health-benefits-antiinflammatory-diet

Hill, A. (2022, July 5). *Eat stop eat review: Does it work for weight loss?* Healthline. https://www.healthline.com/nutrition/eat-stop-eat-review

Hilton Andersen, C. (2019, September 12). *Yes, you can still exercise on an intermittent fasting diet.* Women's Health. https://www.womenshealthmag.com/weight-loss/a29000994/intermittent-fasting-working-out/

Hodges, C. (2019, October 7). *A beginner's guide to meal prep.* EatingWell. https://www.eatingwell.com/article/290651/a-beginners-guide-to-meal-prep/

Holloway, C. (2022, March 3). *Intermittent fasting: 4 different types explained.* Health Essentials from Cleveland Clinic; Health Essentials from Cleveland Clinic. https://health.clevelandclinic.org/intermittent-fasting-4-different-types-explained/

How to use a plant-based diet and intermittent fasting to lose weight. (n.d.). The Beet. Retrieved November 27, 2022, from https://thebeet.com/expert-advice-how-to-use-a-plant-based-diet-and-intermittent-fasting-to-lose-weight/

Howard, B. (2012, October). *What to expect in your 50s - aging, lifestyle, health.* AARP. https://www.aarp.org/health/healthy-living/info-09-2012/what-to-expect-in-your-50s.html

Intermittent fasting: Common myths + FAQ. (n.d.). Christa Biegler. https://www.christabiegler.com/blog/intermittent-fasting-common-myths-faq

Intermittent fasting: What is it, and how does it work? (2022, October 20). John Hopkins Medicine. https://www.hopkinsmedicine.org/health/wellness-and-prevention/intermittent-fasting-what-is-it-and-how-does-it-work

Intermountain Healthcare. (2022, July 7). *People who practice intermittent fasting experience less severe complications from COVID-19, study finds.* ScienceDaily. https://www.sciencedaily.com/releases/2022/07/220707100915.htm

ISSA. (2022, April 1). *Intermittent fasting: Women vs. men.* ISSA. https://www.issaonline.com/blog/post/this-hot-diet-trend-is-not-recommended-for-women

Jhaveri, A., & Felman, A. (2020, April 27). *A vegan-friendly grocery list for anyone going plant based.* Greatist. https://greatist.com/eat/vegan-grocery-list

Johnson, J. (2019, January 28). *The 5:2 diet: A guide and meal plan.* MedicalNewsToday. https://www.medicalnewstoday.com/articles/324303

Kamb, S. (2022, January 1). *Intermittent fasting for beginners: Should you skip breakfast?* Nerd Fitness. https://www.nerdfitness.com/blog/a-beginners-guide-to-intermittent-fasting/

Keefer, A. (2021, March 15). *10 beginner's tips to meal planning like a pro.* Healthy Family Project. https://healthyfamilyproject.com/10-beginners-tips-meal-planning-like-pro/

Keller, C. (2020, December 16). *Make intermittent fasting fit your schedule.* USANA. https://whatsupusana.com/2020/12/intermittent-fasting/

Kriehn, J. (n.d.). *What to eat during intermittent fasting when you socialize.* MyNetDiary. https://www.mynetdiary.com/what-to-eat-during-intermittent-fasting.html

Kubala, J. (2018, July 3). *The warrior diet: Review and beginner's guide.* Healthline; Healthline Media. https://www.healthline.com/nutrition/warrior-diet-guide

Kubala, J. (2020, July 1). *One meal a day diet: Benefits, risks, and more.* Healthline. https://www.healthline.com/health/one-meal-a-day

Kubala, J. (2021, April 23). *9 potential intermittent fasting side effects.* Healthline. https://www.healthline.com/nutrition/intermittent-fasting-side-effects

Kucine, J. (2018, November 8). *Benefits of intermittent fasting.* Dr. Jeff Kucine D.O. https://www.drkucine.com/benefits-of-intermittent-fasting/

Lab, P. (2021, November 9). *Does taking vitamins break a fast? - 6 safe to take and 4 to avoid while fasting.* Performance Lab. https://www.performancelab.com/blogs/multi/does-taking-vitamins-break-a-fast

Lachtrupp, E. (2022, April 28). *Plant-Based meal plan for beginners.* EatingWell. https://www.eatingwell.com/article/7826129/plant-based-meal-plan-for-beginners/

Landsverk, G., & Brueck, H. (2019, December 12). *Google revealed the top trending diet searches of 2019, and it included plans from celebrities like J. Lo and Adele.* Insider. https://www.insider.com/most-popular-diets-2019-intermittent-fasting-noom-google-search-2019-12#1-intermittent-fasting-was-the-no-1-diet-trend-of-the-year-10

Lawler, M. (2020, January 17). *9 scientific benefits of following a plant-based diet.* Everyday Health. https://www.everydayhealth.com/diet-nutrition/scientific-benefits-following-plant-based-diet/

Lawler, M. (2022a, February 10). *12 burning questions about intermittent fasting, answered.* Everyday Health. https://www.everydayhealth.com/diet-nutrition/burning-questions-about-intermittent-fasting-answered/

Lawler, M. (2022b, August 15). *Beginner's guide to a plant-based diet: Food list, meal plan, benefits, and more.* Everyday Health. https://www.everydayhealth.com/diet-nutrition/plant-based-diet-food-list-meal-plan-benefits-more/

Lederer, S. (2021, July 1). *Clean vs. dirty intermittent fasting – which is more effective?* MentalFoodChain. https://www.mentalfoodchain.com/clean-vs-dirty-intermittent-fasting/

Lehnardt, K. (2017, January 9). *74 interesting facts about weight loss.* Fact Retriever. https://www.factretriever.com/weight-loss-facts

Leonard, J. (2020, January 17). *16:8 intermittent fasting: Benefits, how-to, and tips.* Medical News Today. https://www.medicalnewstoday.com/articles/327398

Lindberg, S. (2020, September 1). *How to exercise safely during intermittent fasting.* Healthline. https://www.healthline.com/health/how-to-exercise-safely-intermittent-fasting

Link, R. (2018, September 4). *16/8 intermittent fasting: A beginner's guide.* Healthline; Healthline Media. https://www.healthline.com/nutrition/16-8-intermittent-fasting

Longo, Valter D., & Mattson, Mark P. (2014). Fasting: Molecular mechanisms and clinical applications. *Cell Metabolism, 19*(2), 181–192. https://doi.org/10.1016/j.cmet.2013.12.008

Magee, E. (n.d.). *Foods to help keep your skin healthy.* WebMD. https://www.webmd.com/skin-problems-and-treatments/acne/features/skin-foods

Mann, D. (2022, January 13). *What to know about intermittent fasting for women.* The Healthy. https://www.thehealthy.com/weight-loss/intermittent-fasting-for-women/

Marinac, C. R., Nelson, S. H., Breen, C. I., Hartman, S. J., Natarajan, L., Pierce, J. P., Flatt, S. W., Sears, D. D., & Patterson, R. E. (2016). Prolonged nightly fasting and breast cancer prognosis. *JAMA Oncology, 2*(8), 1049–1055. https://doi.org/10.1001/jamaoncol.2016.0164

Marks, B. (2022, September 5). *Brooke Burke, 50, reveals toned tummy in a crop top while biking.* Mail Online. https://www.dailymail.co.uk/tvshowbiz/article-11180051/Brooke-Burke-50-reveals-toned-tummy-crop-biking-fianc-Scott-Rigsby-Malibu.html

Martinac, P. (2011, May 11). *How eat-stop-eat works.* Livestrong; Livestrong.com. https://www.livestrong.com/article/438695-how-eat-stop-eat-works/

Mathur, K., Agrawal, R. K., Nagpure, S., & Deshpande, D. (2020). Effect of artificial sweeteners on insulin resistance among type-2 diabetes mellitus patients. *Journal of Family Medicine and Primary Care, 9*(1), 69–71. https://doi.org/10.4103/jfmpc.jfmpc_329_19

McAuliffe, L. (2022, August 11). *The 20 hour fast: Benefits and how to.* Dr. Robert Kiltz. https://www.doctorkiltz.com/20-hour-fast/

Mdrive. (2022, February 6). *The guide to 18:6 intermittent fasting.* Mdrive. https://www.mdriveformen.com/blogs/the-driven/18-6-intermittent-fasting-schedule

Mehmet, S. (2021, April 22). *16:8 diet plan: What can you eat and what are the benefits?* GoodtoKnow. https://www.goodto.com/wellbeing/diets-exercise/16-8-diet-plan-289305

Meola, K. (2019, November 22). *Celebrities who swear by intermittent fasting.* Us Weekly. https://www.usmagazine.com/celebrity-body/pictures/intermittent-fasting-diet-trend-celebrity-success-stories/

Migala, J. (2022, February 18). *What is intermittent fasting? A detailed beginner's guide.* Everyday Health. https://www.everydayhealth.com/diet-nutrition/intermittent-fasting/

Millard, E. (2020, July 30). *Trying intermittent fasting? Here's how to choose the right timeframe for you.* Bicycling. https://www.bicycling.com/news/a33444211/best-intermittent-fasting-schedule-for-you-study/

Miller, K. (2021, March 1). *The eat stop eat diet involves fasting for 24 hours at a time.* Women's Health. https://www.womenshealthmag.com/weight-loss/a22689488/eat-stop-eat-diet/

Miller, S. (2022, May 27). *Intermittent fasting and insulin resistance: Benefits beyond weight loss.* Jefferson Health. https://www.jeffersonhealth.org/your-health/living-well/intermittent-fasting-and-insulin-resistance-benefits-beyond-weight-loss

Morales-Brown, L. (2020, June 11). *Intermittent fasting and exercise: How to do it safely.* MedicalNewsToday. https://www.medicalnewstoday.com/articles/intermittent-fasting-and-working-out

Mudge, L. (2022, March 11). *Alternate day fasting: What is it and how does it work?* Live Science. https://www.livescience.com/alternate-day-fasting

National Cancer Institute. (2018, December 16). *Breast cancer risk in American women.* National Cancer Institute; Cancer.gov. https://www.cancer.gov/types/breast/risk-fact-sheet

National Eating Disorders Collaboration. (n.d.). *Disordered eating & dieting.* NEDC. https://nedc.com.au/eating-disorders/eating-disorders-explained/disordered-eating-and-dieting/

Neidler, S. (2022, November 17). *20/4 intermittent fasting: All you need to know.* WeFast. https://www.wefast.care/articles/intermittent-fasting-20-4

Nutrafol Team. (2019, October 11). *Women need to know this before trying intermittent fasting.* Nutrafol. https://nutrafol.com/blog/intermittent-fasting-men-women/

Padley, I. (2022, January 6). *Learn about Jennifer Lopez's intermittent fasting experience.* Fastyle Blog. https://www.fastyle.me/blog/jennifer-lopez-and-intermittent-fasting/

Pahwa, R., & Jialal, I. (2019, June 4). *Chronic inflammation.* NIH; StatPearls Publishing. https://www.ncbi.nlm.nih.gov/books/NBK493173/

Pannell, N. (2018, August 27). *10 things you've heard about intermittent fasting that aren't true.* Insider. https://www.insider.com/intermittent-fasting-myths-2018-8

Panoff, L. (2019, September 26). *What breaks a fast? Foods, drinks, and supplements.* Healthline. https://www.healthline.com/nutrition/what-breaks-a-fast

Parker, K. (2021, June 30). *The effect of intermittent fasting on your brain.* Aviv Clinics USA. https://aviv-clinics.com/blog/nutrition/the-effect-of-intermittent-fasting-on-your-brain/

Pennesi, J.-L., & Wade, T. D. (2016). A systematic review of the existing models of disordered eating: Do they inform the development of effective interventions? *Clinical Psychology Review, 43*, 175–192. https://doi.org/10.1016/j.cpr.2015.12.004

Petre, A. (2018, September 30). *How to meal prep — A beginner's guide.* Healthline; Healthline Media. https://www.healthline.com/nutrition/how-to-meal-prep

Petre, A. (2022, July 12). *Vegan intermittent fasting: Pros, cons, meal plan.* Healthline. https://www.healthline.com/nutrition/vegan-intermittent-fasting

Picard, C. (2020, October 12). *These are calorie counting apps that can actually help you lose weight, according to nutritionists.* Good Housekeeping. https://www.goodhousekeeping.com/health-products/g28246667/best-calorie-counting-apps/

Plowe, K. (2020, December 8). *Complete plant-based diet grocery list.* EatingWell. https://www.eatingwell.com/article/7878282/complete-plant-based-diet-grocery-list/

*Positive attitude about aging could boost health. (2022, August 24). News. https://www.hsph.harvard.edu/news/hsph-in-the-news/positive-attitude-about-aging-could-boost-health/*Prescott, K. (2020, September 11). *Battle lactose intolerance by changing the time you eat.* ILLUMINATION. https://medium.com/illumination/battle-lactose-intolerance-by-changing-the-time-you-eat-d7b3bbc749df

Putka, S. (2021, July 9). *Male and female bodies can respond differently to intermittent fasting.* Inverse. https://www.inverse.com/mind-body/intermittent-fasting-difference-men-women

Renee, J. (2018, November 28). *Diet vs. lifestyle change.* Sfgate. https://healthyeating.sfgate.com/diet-vs-lifestyle-change-11130.html

Richards, L. (2020, December 22). *Everything to know about the warrior diet.* Medical News Today. https://www.medicalnewstoday.com/articles/warrior-diet

Rose, E. (2022, April 1). OMAD: Should you do the one meal a day diet? Bulletproof. https://www.bulletproof.com/diet/intermittent-fasting/omad-one-meal-a-day-diet/

Sachdev, P. (2022, February 22). *9 ways to eat clean.* WebMD. https://www.webmd.com/diet/ss/slideshow-how-to-eat-clean

Salzberg, S. (2020, January 6). *Can intermittent fasting reset your immune system?* Forbes. https://www.forbes.com/sites/stevensalzberg/2020/01/06/can-intermittent-fasting-reset-your-immune-system/?sh=3023014027ac

Siefert, R. (2020, March 2). *Ways you didn't know your body changes after 50.* The Daily Meal. https://www.thedailymeal.com/healthy-eating/body-changes-after-50-gallery

Soeters, M. R., Sauerwein, H. P., Groener, J. E., Aerts, J. M., Ackermans, M. T., Glatz, J. F. C., Fliers, E., & Serlie, M. J. (2007). Gender-related differences in the metabolic response to fasting. *The Journal of Clinical Endocrinology and Metabolism, 92*(9), 3646–3652. https://doi.org/10.1210/jc.2007-0552

Spritzler, F. (2022, January 7). 11 simple ways to start clean eating today. Healthline; Healthline Media. https://www.healthline.com/nutrition/11-ways-to-eat-clean

Stanton, B. (2020, July 31). *7 common intermittent fasting myths, debunked.* HUM Nutrition Blog. https://www.humnutrition.com/blog/intermittent-fasting-myths/#7_Myths_About_Intermittent_Fasting

Stote, K. S., Baer, D. J., Spears, K., Paul, D. R., Harris, G. K., Rumpler, W. V., Strycula, P., Najjar, S. S., Ferrucci, L., Ingram, D. K., Longo, D. L., & Mattson, M. P. (2007). A controlled trial of reduced meal frequency without caloric restriction in healthy, normal-weight, middle-aged adults. *The American Journal of Clinical Nutrition, 85*(4), 981–988. https://doi.org/10.1093/ajcn/85.4.981

Suazo, A. (2022, February 10). *How to meal prep: A beginner's guide for perfect make-ahead meals.* Bulletproof. https://www.bulletproof.com/diet/healthy-eating/how-to-meal-prep-beginners-guide/

Sugar, J. (2021, November 23). *What is the 18:6 intermittent fasting method?* POPSUGAR Fitness. https://www.popsugar.com/fitness/What-186-Intermittent-Fasting-45446501

Supplements - multivitamins. (n.d.). DrFuhrman.com. https://shop.drfuhrman.com/supplements/multivitamins/

Swiner, C. (2021, June 29). *What to expect in your 50s.* WebMD. https://www.webmd.com/healthy-aging/ss/slideshow-what-to-expect-in-your-50s

Tamber, M., & Scher, B. (2022, March 31). *Intermittent fasting (IF): Your complete guide.* Diet Doctor. https://www.dietdoctor.com/intermittent-fasting

Tello, M. (2018, June 26). *Intermittent fasting: Surprising update.* Harvard Health Blog. https://www.health.harvard.edu/blog/intermittent-fasting-surprising-update-2018062914156

10 tips for planning meals on a budget - unlock food. (n.d.). Unlockfood. https://www.unlockfood.ca/en/Articles/Budget/10-Tips-for-Planning-Meals-on-a-Budget.aspx

The Daily Meal Staff. (2020, February 20). *Best teas to settle an upset stomach.* The Daily Meal. https://www.thedailymeal.com/healthy-eating/teas-settle-stomach-gallery

Thompson, S. R. (2021, August 29). *Pregnancy, parenting, lifestyle, beauty: Tips & advice.* MamasLatinas. https://mamaslatinas.com/healthy-you/celebrity-diets-jennifer-lopez-adele/methods-fasting

Tinsley, G. (2017, September 17). *Time-Restricted eating: A beginner's guide.* Healthline; Healthline Media. https://www.healthline.com/nutrition/time-restricted-eating

Toledano, S. (2022, April 12). *What is a plant-based diet, and is it healthy?* Columbia University Irving Medical Center. https://www.cuimc.columbia.edu/news/what-plant-based-diet-and-it-healthy

Trumpfeller, G. (2020, July 22). *Do you need to take supplements during intermittent fasting?* Simple.life Blog. https://simple.life/blog/intermittent-fasting-and-supplements/

Tyler, A. (2022, May 23). *The easy guide to 18:6 intermittent fasting.* Hone Health. https://honehealth.com/edge/nutrition/186-intermittent-fasting

Uher, R., Treasure, J., Heining, M., Brammer, M. J., & Campbell, I. C. (2006). Cerebral processing of food-related stimuli: Effects of fasting and gender. *Behavioural Brain Research, 169*(1), 111–119. https://doi.org/10.1016/j.bbr.2005.12.008

University of New South Wales. (2009, April 4). *Why do women store fat differently from men?* ScienceDaily. https://www.sciencedaily.com/releases/2009/03/090302115755.htm

University of North Carolina at Chapel Hill. (2008, April 23). *Three out of four American women have disordered eating, survey suggests.* ScienceDaily. https://www.sciencedaily.com/releases/2008/04/080422202514.htm

Valente, L. (2022, November 6). *7 tips for clean eating.* EatingWell. https://www.eatingwell.com/article/78846/7-tips-for-clean-eating/

Varady, K. A. (2011). Intermittent versus daily calorie restriction: which diet regimen is more effective for weight loss? *Obesity Reviews, 12*(7), e593–e601. https://doi.org/10.1111/ j.1467-789x.2011.00873.x

Varady, K. A., Cienfuegos, S., Ezpeleta, M., & Gabel, K. (2021). Cardiometabolic benefits of intermittent fasting. *Annual Review of Nutrition, 41*(1), 333–361. https://doi.org/10.1146/annurev-nutr-052020-041327

Vetter, C. (2022a, January 26). *Intermittent fasting for women: Here's what you need to know.* Join Zoe. https://joinzoe.com/learn/intermittent-fasting-for-women

Vetter, C. (2022b, November 2). *Intermittent fasting: What can you eat or drink?* Join Zoe. https://joinzoe.com/learn/what-to-eat-or-drink-while-intermittent-fasting

Waehner, P. (2020, January 21). *4 effective ways to track your weight loss progress.* Verywell Fit. https://www.verywellfit.com/ways-to-track-weight-loss-progress-1231581

Wahi, S. (2020, December 16). *Everything Halle Berry did to get the body she has today.* Marie Claire. https://www.marieclaire.com.au/halle-berry-exercise-routine

Walton, C. (2022, July 29). *Intermittent fasting for women over 50: Benefits and tips for success.* Better Weigh Medical. https://betterweighmedical.com/intermittent-fasting-for-women-over-50

Warren, S. (2022, August 12). *The health benefits of multi-day and intermittent fasting.* Somatic Movement Center. https://somaticmovementcenter.com/intermittent-fasting/?locale=en

Waterhouse, J. (2020, October 16). *9 celebrities who swear by intermittent fasting.* Marie Claire. https://www.marieclaire.com.au/intermittent-fasting-celebrities

Weingus, L. (2021, April 21). *Is intermittent fasting safe for women? It's complicated, so here's how to set yourself up for IF success.* Parade. https://parade.com/1064585/leighweingus/intermittent-fasting-for-women/

Wellness & Prevention. (2022, June 7). *What is insulin resistance weight gain?* Scripps Health. https://www.scripps.org/news_items/4621-can-insulin-resistance-cause-weight-gain

Wisdom, E. (2022, January 11). *Taking supplements while intermittent fasting: All you need to know.* Earth's Wisdom. https://earths-wisdom.com/blogs/wisdom-news/taking-supplements-while-intermittent-fasting-all-you-need-to-know

Woods, L. (2021, January 25). *Intermittent fasting and working out: Here's what science actually says about this combo.* BetterMe Blog. https://betterme.world/articles/intermittent-fasting-and-working-out/

Working out while intermittent fasting. (n.d.). Akins. https://www.atkins.com/how-it-works/library/articles/6-things-to-know-about-intermittent-fasting-and-working-out

Yeager, S. F., Heim, R., Seile, J., & Lofton, H. (2008). *Self-Monitoring - the way to successful weight management.* Obesity Action Coalition. https://www.obesityaction.org/resources/self-monitoring-the-way-to-successful-weight-management/

Made in the USA
Las Vegas, NV
02 December 2024

13210086R00174